Other titles by **SHARNY ⦿ JULIUS**

PREG FIT

HOW I FINALLY HAD A FIT, HEALTHY, HAPPY **PREGNANCY** AND **PAIN FREE** BIRTH

SHARNY ⚭ JULIUS
www.sharnyandjulius.com

PregFIT by SHARNY ✄ JULIUS

How I finally had a fit, healthy, happy pregnancy and pain free birth

www.sharnyandjulius.com
email:sharnyandjulius@sharnyandjulius.com

Copyright © the Kieser Publishing Trust
First published by Kieser Publishing Trust in Nov 2014

Edited by:	Laura Hawkskin McGawkskin Johnno Johnson AKA Miss Cessnock; mother of much talent and courage.
Front Cover Photography:	sharnyandjulius
Back Cover Photography:	Captured by Bec
Typesetting and Design:	sharnyandjulius
ISBN:	978-0-9923613-1-0

Contents

You've got this

Emmett, my second youngest son, is happy. Happy all the time. But not just any kind of happy, he's distracted happy. He's distracted by happiness.

If Alexis and Danté (his older siblings, but not by much) are fighting next to him, he notices, but doesn't engage; he just smiles, watches for a bit, then looks away into the distance, as though he is listening to another voice, a voice inside his little head that must be whispering the most magical, beautiful things. The look on his face is distracted with what can only be described as a *knowing* smile.

It's as though he knows something nobody else knows. Like we've won the lottery and he's the only one who knows it. The rest of us hustle through our days making the most of them, but he knows, he just knows that everything will be awesome.

Emmett is a calming, beautiful person to be around.

I had my first baby Josh when I was only 16. I was only a child and felt like (and was told) that I had done the wrong thing. The entire birthing experience echoed my inner fears. 36 hours of labour and he was finally dragged out. After that immensely stressful, horrendous ordeal; I swore I'd never ever have any more kids.

But here I am. Only a few weeks after birth number 5. This one's name is Hugo. Alexis and Danté talked to Hugo when he was just a baby bump. Often, they go out of their way to give my belly a little kiss. It's moments like those that make me grateful that I never let my fears get the better of me all those years ago.

It did take me a while though. Josh was 14 years old when we decided that we would expand the family. "Don't do it!" Our friends would say, "You're nearly free!". I laugh now and think, what is free, when you have nobody to share it with.

Julius and I want a huge family. We decided 5 was our number. Maybe it was because Julius comes from a family of 4 and he is competitive, or maybe it is because 5 was just the right number for us. Whatever the reason, we'd settled into the idea that we were going to have 5 kids.

But Alexis kept saying to me; "Mummy, after Hugo comes out of your fanny, we'll get a girl; OK?"

6 kids? We'll see.

Joshua's birth was insane; but each subsequent birth just got better. Partly because I got a bit of practice, but mostly because I didn't want a repeat performance. It scared me.

And that, is the problem.

Fear.

The overriding outcome of you reading this book is that you eradicate fear. Not eliminate, eradicate. Fear is the single greatest risk to a pregnancy.

Julius explains it in an overly simple man-way;

It's like standing at the urinal when I'm about to pee. Next thing a guy stands right next to me. You can feel how close he is. He gets his junk out and I haven't even started yet. Like a fountain he lets his tide go. Splashing all up on my shoes, I can feel my pee hole begin to close up. "Nope, not today," it says. But further up the water works, we've opened the floodgates. The pressure is immense, in my head I'm thinking "I'm like an old guy with kidney stones."

The whole time the stranger next to me is peeing, I'm standing there with my dick in my hand. The next thought that comes into my head is "push". I can't have someone start after me and finish before me. Forget what I'm thinking; he's probably wondering what the hell I'm doing. Standing there, dry cock in hand; face glowing like a stop sign and nothing to show for it.

Every effort to push only serves to close the pee hole even tighter. It's starting to really hurt. For some reason I care (and I wish I didn't but I do) what Mr Nobody thinks of me. And it tightens the pee hole even more. Then one of two things happens. Either I dribble a token little bit of pee on my shoes (which starts the fear cycle again) or I pop a quick shart.

Shart? Shit fart. When the pressure is so much that you pass more than just wind.

It is at this point that I just pack my dribbly little dick up and go sit on the toilet like a girl.

What I was afraid of all the time.

This may be simple and funny, but it is exactly what makes birth go wrong.

Fear. Fear that it is going to go wrong, brings about that very thing. Fear closes the exit hole. Fear tightens the perineum and reduces blood flow to the birthing muscles. Fear speeds the heart rate and floods the system with adrenalin. Before you know it, your body is pushing against itself. The top half is pushing down, but the bottom half doesn't want the baby to come.

And it's natural.

It's a natural response. Imagine a deer giving birth in the quiet of a tree. All of a sudden it hears a wolf howl. If it gives birth now, both mother and fawn will be eaten. Fear stops the process. Being in a hospital bed, surrounded by white coat men who talk about you, not to you, sparks fear. Friends telling you horror stories, sparks fear. Movies depicting women screaming "you did this to me!" sparks fear.

Seeing a birth doctor, birthing in the hospital, you can be forgiven for getting the feeling that birth is a medical emergency. A medical emergency is terrifying.

Fear makes painful births. Fear makes stressful births. Fear breeds fear.

Let's eradicate fear.

Let's be more like Emmett.

Because you are.

He knows that he's got this. To a little baby, life is all about experiences, adventure. As we grow older, life becomes one of avoiding danger. We think all the time about "what could go wrong". Emmett doesn't. His entire life is ahead of him, and he doesn't stress about it. Because he's got this. Birth, live a life of maximum experience, then die.

That's pretty much it.   Add any more complexity to it, and you have expectations. Expectations may or may not be met. This alone breeds fear. Emmett has no fear. You should have no fear.

Why?

Because you've got this.

Animals give birth without help.

African women give birth by themselves against a tree, then immediately go back to work. They don't need medical intervention. Medical help is good in case something goes wrong. Not, because birthing is wrong.

You've got this.

And with that, lets get into it.

By the end of this book, I want you to feel like Emmett looks. Happy. Everyone else around you could be shouting and screaming and stressing and fighting, your finances could be going to shit, your body could be falling apart, your husband could be leaving you, the world could be collapsing, the sky falling; but you... you're in your bubble of joy. You... you're distracted by happiness.

Why?

Because you've got this.

You were born for this.

You, and your baby, already know what to do.

What you should get from this book

I've been asked by so many mums to be; "Do you have a fitness program for pregnant mums?"

So the first outcome of the book is to mitigate your loss of fitness.

You see, growing another human inside you takes a lot from you. You know when you're in the shower, and someone turns on the bathroom tap? You're not getting the same amount of water as you're used to, and chances are you're not getting the temperature you'd like.

There's nothing you can do to change it, you can't get more water; you just have to wait or adapt.

Pregnancy is the same. Your baby is the one controlling the bathroom tap. You're not. For me, this was a big lesson and a big thing to come to terms with. For 9 months, I am a vessel. I do not control the energy flow. My baby takes what it wants, and leaves me with the rest. I have to adapt. I am not in control.

It is all but impossible to increase your fitness while pregnant. Intensity is what makes fitness, and intensity is what potentially harms you or your baby. So to tell you that you can get fitter while pregnant is misleading.

What you can do, is mitigate your loss of fitness.

Most mums, when they first fall pregnant, realise that they can't get fitter so just make the decision to say "fark that. I'll get fit again once I've had the baby."

Please don't do that to yourself.

One of the worst things you can do to yourself is to give up and become a breeding sow. You know those pigs who just breed and breastfeed. The farmer doesn't even let them up; they just lay on their sides for years, birthing and feeding, birthing and feeding. Don't be that.

I did it, I'm sure you've got plenty of friends who did it. Maybe your last pregnancy you did it. Don't do it. Fight that urge to give up. Here are a few reasons why it is bad to give up on your health and fitness while pregnant:

- In less than 9 months, you will be fat and unfit.
- You will no longer have the excuse of carrying a baby.
- Time to exercise will be absolutely non existent, all you'll want to do is sleep. Which you can't do.
- Fit healthy mums make fit healthy births and fit healthy children.
- Giving birth is like running a marathon. The energy needs are huge, the stress on the body is immense. Marathons are easy if you are trained, prepared and ready for one. Marathons are all but impossible if you spend 9 months leading up to one "eating for two," or smashing back pies and coke because it's

"what the baby is craving."

Don't do it to yourself. It's only 9 months. Some of it will be hard, but the work you put in now will pay you back ten fold once the baby comes out. Being fit and healthy during pregnancy will make you:

- Able to handle the endurance of a long birth.
- Have supple, flexible joints for a faster, easier birth.
- Pass less stress to the baby during childbirth (makes a much calmer baby).
- Able to bounce back after pregnancy fast.
- Have energy when the baby is born.

In 9 months, you can lose a lot of fitness. You can also gain a lot of weight. The first purpose of this book is to reduce the loss of fitness, because you just can't do some of the things you could sans baby. You will lose some fitness, but we want to make sure that you only lose a little. We want to mitigate the loss of fitness.

The second outcome is that I want you to be fully prepared to bounce back after the birth. Pregnancy and birth is like going on a holiday. You get the most wonderful, indulgent feelings and experiences and you get to learn about yourself in a way you didn't imagine possible.

While you're pregnant, it consumes your every thought. But once the baby is born, life goes on. Life must go on. The holiday is over. Did you spend the time wisely, or did you spend the whole holiday at the buffet?

You know what I'm talking about right? We've been on a holiday once where all we did was eat. Like cattle, we just destroyed the buffet, breakfast, lunch and dinner. "Stuff it, we're on holiday!" we laughed. After the most audacious breakfast, we'd lay by the pool like a pack of fat lions, waiting for the lunch buffet. Gut stretched, mouth slippery. "Stuff it, we're on holiday!" Gluttonous eating like this is hard work, so we'd sleep in the breeze and when we got too hot, we'd plop into the pool like lizards; then straight back to the daybed to order a cocktail.

We were in Fiji. On an island. We could have spent the days fishing, sailing, exploring, discovering the culture. We came back from that holiday fat, tired and no better off. Holidays are a time to better yourself, get some perspective, relax a little.

We came back from that holiday broke and fat. We could have come back from that holiday fitter, enlightened, more cultured and enthused.

Your pregnancy has to end. Once it does, you will never be the same again. Your life will be forever changed. You will have another human to care for. Tied to you forever. You will be a mother. Someone will be soon calling you "mum."

Don't be fooled into thinking that pregnancy and birth are the event. They are like an orientation to mothering. Pregnancy lasts for 9 months, mothering lasts forever. It is the greatest gift you could ever receive. The unbridled love and trust of another human being.

You have to do everything in your power to make that life one worth living. Bounce back fast, be the greatest mother that ever lived. You know you can. You know you will.

The third, and most important outcome of this book is for you to have an empowering birth.

Bouncing back is important, but it's not worth stressing yourself over. Right now, you are pregnant. Right now, you are growing a baby inside of you. You are doing something that half the population can never do. You are doing something completely impossible.

Childbirth is an absolute miracle, and you are the one who gets to go through it. For 9 months, you get to experience the most amazing, empowering, delightful, self-fulfilling thing you could probably ever do.

Growing a baby inside you is like a holiday of enlightenment. When you decided to skip the buffet and walk outside, you'll get this wonderful sense of adventure. It seems that every day with every pregnancy, I learn something about myself. About the world. About the world inside myself.

While the world hustles by, you are on a spiritual journey inside your mind and inside your body. No man can ever do what you are doing. They have to conquer mountains and swim across oceans, or walk on coals to get even a tiny snippet of the power you have coursing through you right now. Take a moment to feel it.

Put your hands on your tummy and breathe really, really slowly. Deep. In and out. Close your eyes for a minute and feel it. The energy inside you. The energy within you. The energy surrounding you.

People call it a pregnancy glow. Scientists call is hormones. I just like to believe that I have been given a gift of enlightenment. A God, somewhere believes I am responsible enough to be given another human to care for, for the rest of his/her life.

They say a woman is reborn with her child. You may feel like you just want the baby out and the pregnancy to be over, but 9 months goes so fast. Before you know it, this will be all over and the only thing left will be the memory.

Will you have a painful, fearful memory; or will you have an empowering, enlightening memory. When you say "In those 9 months, my entire life changed," will it be for the better, or the worse. The choice is yours. You DO have a choice.

Who am I?

My name is Sharny, I have written a few books and have 5 kids. I have one brother and no biological sisters. But what I do have is a connection to thousands and thousands of women. Like sisters. Soul sisters.

Not to be confused with soul *sistas*. I have no rhythm and my wedding dance looked like a puppet show. For 5 whole minutes, Julius and I fought with the rusty hinges of our rigid bodies to attempt a wedding waltz. ONE, two, three... ONE, two, three.

No, not much soul in this sister; but I feel like I have ten thousand sisters. It's hard to explain it to a man, because they don't really understand the bond between girls. Julius kind of gets it; he's got 2 brothers (there are 3 years between the three of them) and they share a very tight bond.

I feel that when I meet and talk to another mum or mum to be, or read the comments on my blog or social media, or the excited OMG's and tons of exclamation marks when one of you gorgeous girls gets to a goal, or overcomes a previously insurmountable obstacle.

"OMG!!! I did it!!!!!"

I love my sisters; together, we really show the power of community, of reaching out. Of sisterhood.

So think of me as a sister. Not older, not younger, not wiser. Just a sister who has gone through 5 births and learnt a few things along the way.

Please don't think of me as an expert or a guru. There are plenty of women who are better at birth than me, and plenty with bigger qualifications. Again, there are plenty of mums with far more kids than I. I am nobody special, and nobody to look up to; all I am is a mother with a unique perspective. What you read in these chapters works for me, but if you feel like it won't work for you, don't worry - just discard it.

Do what is right for you.

Closet Obstetricians

How do you know someone is Vegan? Don't worry. *They* will tell you.

It's the same with pregnancy, except backwards. How do you know you're pregnant? Don't worry, everyone will tell you.

Pregnancy is like religion and politics. Everybody has a very strong opinion that they think is right. No, let's go one step further; they *believe* is right. And they don't mind Shoving. It. Down. Your. Throat.

The same thing happened the first time we went on TV. Everyone around us, suddenly became a TV interview expert. "You should say this, don't do this, sit like this, I wouldn't do that. Whatever you do, don't do this. Make sure you do that." On and on and on. All the closet TV experts made us feel overwhelmed. By the time we got to our interview, we were both so nervous and worried about all the things we were meant to say and do, that we nearly froze.

It's the same with pregnancy. Before falling pregnant, you just thought the people around you were normal, living normal lives.

How wrong you were.

It turns out; most people are actually *pretending* to be normal. Like superheroes.

You'll probably know it by now, but in case you hadn't noticed; the world is filled with closet obstetricians. Who would have thought!

Even the ladies at the supermarket have obstetrics degrees. I'm convinced that once you're pregnant, you get a sign on your head that reads "I need all the help I can get." You can't read it of course, I mean, you're the one having the baby, what could you possibly know anyway, but by god it must be there; every closet obstetrician or midwife is there to offer advice.

And it's free. Not even bulk billed!

Where we live, there is a footpath along the beachfront that people use to get fit. It's a beautiful walk up over the hill overlooking the ocean; people running by joyfully.

Once, I was walking along behind the kids while Julius pushed Emmett in his pram and they rode their little bikes, when the garbage guy looks up at me, wheelie bin in hand and says "It's a girl! Definitely a girl." Amazing, an obstetrician doing some community service. Unheard of. "I can tell," he continued, "never been wrong before!"

Why go to church to find God, when you can find him in the hospital? There is this ego that surgeons have that they are God like. Julius' family is all medical; they all know it and joke about it. There is this common idea in hospitals that surgeons are pretty much Gods. Obestricians are a type of surgeon.

So here I am, walking along the beach, and I meet a man-god surgeon, who not only knows how to tell the sex of the baby, but has an MRI machine *inside his head.*

"Make sure you take your folate tablets young lady," the lovely doctor finishes as he climbs into his truck.

You could just take the advice. Everybody actually means well, but after a while (the first real week) it can get quite tiring and confusing. When I say first real week, it is the week when people are convinced you're actually pregnant, not just getting fat.

It turns out that these miracle pro-bono doctors didn't all go to the same medical school. One of them will tell you to take folate because without it, your baby will die, and the next is adamant that folate is pharmaceutical profiteering that will kill your baby. *Kill* your baby. These words are very powerful, it's no wonder we're scared.

A baby is so precious, so helpless, so fragile, we know. WE BLOODY WELL KNOW!!

But it's up to us; Mum. Nobody else to make the decisions that sit best with us and our child. Nobody else.

Even the real obstetricians are not so sure.

The first two kids of mine had a different blood type to me. My obstetrician told me that I had to take an anti D injection to ensure that the baby's immune system didn't turn against me in the womb. Scary. So I took the injections and when it came time for that conversation with Danté my third, the same obstetrician said "We've done research and it's proven more risky so we won't be giving you your anti D injections."

Here's the deal.

Everybody may well be an expert. But only you can push the baby out.
Only you can carry the baby. Only you will be caring for the baby once
it comes out. You are in charge. You know what's best. You are the
mother. Own that. It's a title for life.

Like sportsmen and critics. Critics can sit in the stands and yell abuse,
have expert opinions, have logical arguments. But none of them are in
the game. They're watching. Athletes don't listen to critics. They choose
coaches and mentors, and that's it.

Coaches and mentors are sounding boards. They cannot play the game
for you. You're in the game. You're the lead role in this play.

Naysayers

The next step down from the closet doctor is the doom and gloom naysaying story teller.

"... you heard about that woman and her baby that died only last week because she was allergic to, like cat hair and by breathing it in, she infected her baby and the next day she's on the toilet right, and when she's finished with what she thinks is a big poo, and looks into the toilet to find her baby lying there looking up at her all like *"mummy, you killed me"*.

What?

Seriously, what?

What can I do with a story like that. What can I learn? What can I possibly ever benefit from such a terrifying, horrific story. Why do you even feel like telling it to me? Who the fuck are you?

But all I can muster is an "Oh, wow..."

This story above is real. It was told to me by a woman at a gala dinner. Some stories you can't even unhear.

But this happens more than any mother would like to imagine. As if it isn't scary enough, we've got the doomsday naysayers who feel it is their place to tell you their horror story. I swear I've heard them all, everyone has a scary as hell story to tell that involves death, disease, blood and birth.

And the ones who tell you their horror story like they are proud? "I was in labour for like, 57 hours straight. The doctors cut me from asshole to throat. I had 15 kids in there."

What they're saying between the lines is:

"you're gonna get messed up in there. It's a right of passage. No pain no gain!" I picture these psychos punching their guts before pregnancy to prepare themselves for the ordeal. And when it's over, they're going to tell the world. I'm surprised there isn't a shirt with "I survived childbirth" printed on it. Flip the shirt over and you have a checklist of all the horrible things you can tick off.

Premature baby: tick!

Massive blood loss: tick!

Third world country: tick!

Baby nearly died: tick!

I nearly died: tick!

Labour duration: _____ days

Emergency cesarian: tick!

Shat myself: ...um, no

That last one is a lie. Everybody shits themselves. Nobody likes to admit it, but how can you not shit yourself. Both exit holes are so close. In childbirth, you've got to relax downstairs and push from above. Nobody on earth can relax the vagina, but squeeze the anus to a tight seal. Try it now - tighten your coit up real tight, like you've got one of those rogue farts pushing down on it. Now keep that thing locked up while you relax the front. Impossible.

A little bit of poo? Don't stress about that. Most of the time you're told that a curry will bring the baby on. Curry, loose cheeks, big baby?

All you need now is a water birth.

By the time you're done, your bath is gonna look like a Tom Yum Goong. The midwife's eyes are going to be burning from the curry as she sweeps the pool for chunks.

Seriously, this is the only real horror story. Come to terms with the fact that you will very likely shit yourself in front of some strangers, and the rest is just easy peasy soul sista!

When Mrs Horror-Story starts up, especially if it's in a group - Mrs Horror-Story loves an audience. The bigger the better.

When she starts up, as she's taxiing down that runway of "I'm the toughest mutha out there" you could cut her off with the pragmatic "If it's a horror story, I don't want to hear it." But I prefer a more guerilla approach.

"With my first baby, I had the worst birth experience..." when you hear this, cut right in with "did you poo yourself?"

Shoot that airplane down before it even takes off. That's a flight you just don't need to take. Red faced, Mrs Horror-Story will walk away or change the subject. You'll notice too, everybody around her like a pack of vampires waiting for blood, will dissipate embarrassed; but as they walk away you'll notice that they are walking funny. That's because their own cheeks are tightened right up...

Nobody has ever shat themselves...

True story.

My Story

Have you ever been suddenly woken up in the middle of a deep sleep? I mean trance like sleep, where the dream you're having is so vivid, so real that you actually believe it. It's obviously a dream, but it could be so fantastic that you just want to believe it. Or it could be so scary that you want to escape, but can't.

For a whole week, I had this recurring dream. I found myself inside one of the croc cages at the zoo, wading past this enormous crocodile with one of my kids. The dream version of myself was daring, brave and somewhat crazy. I was in there out of choice. I had jumped the fence with Alexis, and we were talking to the crocodile. Teasing it, goading it to come at us. Which it did, but we were fast and could get away.

On and on the dream would go. Get in one side of the pond, and wade slowly past the head of the croc and down the length of it's body and out the other side. For what seemed like hours, we'd do this. Laughing at the croc, teasing it.

Then, at the same time in the dream, I'd be distracted by a chainsaw starting up, or a lawnmower, or a big truck starting right next to the cage. In the exact moment that my attention would shift to the sound, the croc would lunge at me.

There are different versions of the ending to this dream. The first few times, I woke up immediately, sweating and panting. Terrified. But after a few more times, I'd try and stay in the dream a little longer to see if I got away.

I did, just. Well, I got out of the water and started running for the fence. I'd scream for Alexis to run with me, which she would. Much faster than me. In the dream I'd turn around and the crocodile would be out of the water.

At the zoo, they say that a croc out of water is slow. In my nightmare, the croc would grow legs like a human and start full sprinting to me. A powerful Olympic sprinter with a tail and huge gnashing teeth and a roar as distracting as the chainsaw was.

I'd look down and see that in my hands was a toddler. Heavy and slowing me down. The fence was too far away and too high for me to get away from the croc-man. "Roarrr" and I'd be awake.

When I'd calmed down enough to slip back to sleep, I'd be back in the madness of my dream. Getting to this point would happen quicker every time, sometimes I'd just go straight back to the point that I noticed the toddler in my arms. But then everything would go in slow motion. Many times I'd be so angry at myself for being so irresponsible, why would I take a toddler into a croc cage, why would I wade past a croc with a toddler in my arms?

Why would I wade past a croc!!!

"Roarrr" and I'd be awake.

Sometimes I'd get to the fence, sometimes I'd get part way up the fence before I woke up, sometimes I'd throw the toddler over the fence, but I always woke up before the croc got me. His guttural roar got me out of the nightmare.

After a few days, I worked out that Julius was snoring. The sound of the roar was actually him snoring like an old smoker with a chin like a bullfrog. I kicked him every time I'd wake up and tell him to stop snoring. A couple minutes later I'd be back with the croc, close to the fence and he'd roar.

Awake again, I'd give him a shove and go back to sleep. On and on the process would run until I shoved at him, only to find he wasn't there. I couldn't hear him, so I went looking for him and found him fast asleep on the lounge.

"Good!" I thought in my sweaty panicky broken sleep nightmare induced state and went back to bed.

"Roarrr"

I started getting really scared, because I only heard the roar when I was asleep. Something was messing with me. I believe in ghosts and spirits (I'm terrified of them) so I assumed one was here, so kept myself awake, safe under the covers but hot. And so loud. Focussing on keeping the sound of my breathing down so the ghosts wouldn't notice me (because the covers makes me invisible), I'd slip into sleep.

"Roaar!"

On and on it would go, until in a state of utter shock, like an ice bucket to the head, I heard the roar while I was awake. I didn't even breathe for about a minute, because I was so scared.

It. Was. Me!

I was snoring. Snoring!

Snoring like an old smoker with a bullfrog chin. I got straight up and went to the mirror. I was snoring. *But I'm a young woman,* I thought. Only big fat men snore. What I saw in the mirror shocked me.

Sometimes you don't notice something that is staring you straight in the face, it's so obvious yet you just don't see it. Well, standing in the half light of early morning, I was it. I had become obese. I had the bullfrog chin. Hell, I had the tuckshop arms and the double trunk.

But I've been eating clean, I thought. All those hungry mornings, all that exercise. What was going on. And why hadn't I noticed it?

I had found myself in a familiar place. I had become obese without noticing. My power of denial was so strong that I didn't notice 30 kilos going on in about 6 months. 30 kilograms of fat. It was everywhere. Packed around my face, under my chin, on my ass, thighs and on my back. Obviously there was a lot more, there was even fat in my throat, blocking my windpipe while I slept.

Alone in my bathroom, holding onto chunks of fat in the moonlight was more terrifying than the crocodile dream. "You can't be fat, Sharny" I said to myself. "You, I mean… you!" I'd arrogantly believed that because I was a fitness trainer, I'd not get fat.

Boy was I wrong. The fat woman looking at me was so much bigger than the one from yesterday. She looked so sad too. So tired, beady eyes hidden behind mounds of fat on her flush, swollen face.

I stared long and hard at the woman in the mirror, trying to get a grip on what was going on. "I couldn't be fat, I eat healthy" I kept repeating. Every morning I had a smoothie. I remember being hungry a lot. "I've basically been dieting," I said to myself.

All the stress of the dreams as well as the realization I had become obese had worked me up a mighty appetite. I stumbled to the kitchen, too sick to eat I just sat down.

I sat there until Alexis woke up and asked for food. My morning sickness was so strong that I thought I might vomit. I opened a punnet of choc chip cookies and broke off a little bite of one while I made her breakfast. Just a bite, to get rid of the morning sickness.

While I fed her, I snapped off another piece of cookie. *Julius' favourite*, I thought. *Anzac biscuits*. I reached into the punnet for one more, only to find it empty. I was dry, so I drank a big glass of milk. Then another. This one with Alexis. *It's healthy milk, it hasn't been pasteurized or homogenized*, I reassured myself.

I reached into the pack again. *Empty*, I thought; distracted by fickle thoughts. My hand explored the inside of the punnet just to be sure. Just one more bite should clear this morning sickness right up; then I can have breakfast and start my day.

Eggs, tomatoes, bacon, mushrooms. I was salivating while I compiled my breakfast list. My stomach reminded me that I was sick, and my roving hand reminded me that I had eaten the last biscuit.

Biscuit.

Biscuit?

But the box said choc chip *cookies*. I looked up to see that indeed I had been eating Anzac biscuits. *That's weird,* I thought as I looked at the box to be sure. The label said Anzac biscuits.

Damn, I thought. I'd eaten the one and only Anzac biscuit. Getting up to start my breakfast, I tossed the punnet into the trash. As I threw it, I noticed another one in there.

Then it hit me. I had opened and eaten an entire punnet of choc chip cookies, thrown it out, got a new pack of biscuits, this time Anzacs, and eaten that entire packet within about 15 minutes.

I had just wanted one bite. To get rid of the morning sickness.

The fat bitch that was living inside me had made me forget the 30 or 40 biscuits I had eaten between the first and last bite. I opened the fridge to get the eggs out and saw the milk. I had drunk a litre of that too. On the shelf above the eggs was an open packet of chocolate.

I watched my hand dart out, snap a row off and shove it into my mouth. I had it swallowed before I could stop myself. My hand was half way back to the packet (one more row while I prep breakfast) when I froze.
I had become obese without noticing.

I had cheated on myself. The fat woman living inside me was out of control. She was cunning, and gluttonous and had an unending appetite for junk food.

For the next few months, I watched myself eating uncontrollably. I watched myself swell. I refused to leave the house, and my self loathing had me give up on eating anything healthy. I'd start with junk and end with junk. I was sick all day, and all I could do was eat. Consume. Feed.

Giving birth was a blur, the next 3 months were a whirlwind of feeding Danté, lack of sleep and shoveling more shit into my mouth. I had a gym, I was the face of a gym – a picture of me was on the side of my car, but I hadn't been in there for over a year.

I pulled the stickers off one night so that I wouldn't be reminded of who I once had been. I hated myself. I was tired, I was angry, I was hungry and most of all, I hated the woman I was. How dare she think it would be easy. How dare she feel bad about her stretch marks or her tiny boobies. That bitch had no idea how lucky she was.

Somehow, I fell pregnant again, anther distraction to keep me from realizing I was on the food train. My whole life revolved around food and babies. I was pregnant with 2 under 2, so I did the only thing I was good at, I ate.

By the time Emmett was born, I had no idea who I was anymore. I used to have a flat stomach, but I was now round. The hole from where my belly button ring once went stared at me, stretched like a comet. The only way I could get to those pesky ingrowns around my vagina was with a mirror.

One of the friendly ladies at our local woolies said to me one day "You can't have long to go." Emmett was 2 weeks old already. I got into my car and cried for about an hour and decided that enough was enough. Flicking the crumbs off my chest, I made up my mind.

"I am going to do something for me. Anything, except eat junk." My baby was restless all the time and I knew it was because of the garbage he was getting from my breastmilk.

I left all the junk in the trolley and drove off.

When I got home, I asked Julius to get me a whole bunch of different vegetables. Clear the crap out of the cupboards and leave only vegetables. When the veggies arrived, I realized how much I had missed them.

All the food I had been eating was lacking any nutrition, which is what I was hungry for, so after pigging out on vegetables for a few days, my nutrition stabilized and I was not hungry any more. The fog that clouded my mind lifted and I saw clearly again. I wrote my journey into a book, which you will know as *Fit, Healthy, Happy Mum*.

I lost all my excess weight fast, and by the time I fell pregnant with Hugo, I was looking the best I had my entire life. I swore I would not go back to that girl. I would control myself this pregnancy.

I didn't want to go back to being that girl. I wanted a dream pregnancy and birth. Surely, being my 5th, I was allowed one good one.

On the 7th July, after 9 months of the most amazing, liberating pregnancy, I got my dream. A pain free home birth. A healthy, content little boy with glistening eyes and who breastfed easily.

All my previous babies were fussy on the boob. Hugo is not. I can only put it down to my nutrition. Not only food, but my mind. The food I've been feeding my mind.

When I was preg*fat*, I hated myself and told myself constantly. Now that I've been preg*fit*, I can't imagine why I thought everything was so hard. I feel privileged. I feel lucky, like how people who move away from the city just don't get why they worried about traffic before.

Having a healthy pregnancy is a matter of choice. It really is that simple.

And I'm going to show you how. Because you know what? You deserve to know. Every mum deserves to know how to be healthy. In body and in mind. You're doing something many people can't. Bringing up children is rewarding work, but it's hard. We want our kids to grow up happy and unhindered.

How can we do that, if we ourselves are so self loathing. So hateful.

It's that easy. Exercise and eating healthy doesn't work if you hate it. If you feel like you are punishing yourself.

Anlong Pi

Whenever I'm feeling a little pissy about how tough my life is, I think about the people of Anlong Pi.

Anlong Pi is in a place called Siem Reap in Cambodia. It's only a few km from the world famous Angkor temples. Anlong Pi is home to about 300 people, many of which are children.

I first heard about it when I was having a particularly stressful day. I had just found out that Telstra had taken extra money from our account which overdrew it, and the pleasurable people at my bank decided to do the right thing by us and charge us a $35 overdrawn fee.

Emmett was sick with a tummy bug and Alexis was in a mood that made everyone on edge. I discovered later, to my horror that she projects my moods. Even if I'm not in the room, having an argument or feeling just shitty with the world, she picks up on it and behaves the same… Talk about a gut check!

But that's not what this story is about.

I was having a horrible day. The kids were being difficult, Emmett was pooing every half hour and to top it off, both he and Danté were constantly crying. I swear my neighbours hate us or think that our kids are being abused in some way. On a day like this, it's as if they never stop crying.

I was on the phone to Telstra, waiting for the third person I had been transferred to, to decide what to do, or to look it up, or to have a big laugh while I sat there wasting time with them.

I sat in front of the computer to log into my banking and got distracted, as I do. Julius tells me I have a short attention span, but when I'm pregnant, I'm like that fish off *Finding Nemo*. So I sat down to check the banking and somehow got lost in the internet and came to a page showcasing this place called Anlong Pi.

I'll try to describe it, but I can't do it justice. So I suggest you just Google it and look at the pictures yourself. Anlong Pi *is* a dump. Not in the figurative sense we say when we look at house after a few too many days of missed cleaning. Anlong Pi is a dump. A refuse tip. Garbage trucks pull up and empty the city's trash into the tip.

Unlike our Western refuse tips, this place is home to people. Families. Women and children live in the tip every day scrounging for food. The photos are so confronting. Children with no shoes, bent over in the garbage, digging for food scraps to eat.

When the garbage trucks arrive, the people crowd around them to get first pickings. Think about what you put into your wheelie bin. Nappies, food scraps, broken glass. Everything you don't want gets thrown in the bin and taken away.

I gag if I catch a whiff of the wheelie bin, and the most disgusting thing that has ever happened to me was getting some bin juice on my shoes. And it's my own garbage. In Anlong Pi dump, these families trawl through that garbage every single day. They don't even escape it to go to sleep, because they sleep on the dump, covered by garbage. There are no showers there, and they can't wash their hands. They just dig through the garbage until the find something edible and pop it straight into their mouths.

The children, some only 2 or 3 years old, spend all day collecting potential food in old containers and plastic bags and bringing it to their pregnant mothers. That's right, mothers give birth on the dump. There is no sterilisation, no doctor, no pain killers, they just give birth naturally in the middle of a dump.

When I read this, my eyes welled up with tears. And to see the photos of the children will give you chills down your spine as well as a new perspective on how lucky we truly are.

We will never know the poverty of these people. They will never learn to read, and will grow up on the dump, unwashed and filthy, have sex for the first time with another dump occupant. Obviously they won't have protection, so they'll give birth to the next generation of dump dwellers.

I sat there for a long time with the Telstra on-hold music playing monotonously through the screams of my children thinking only that I was the luckiest woman on earth.

One photo in the collection haunts me every time I feel like being a spoilt little princess. A boy, about 6 years old holds an broken styrofoam container. Inside the Styrofoam container is a clear plastic bag with blackish red congealed mess inside it. The boy has a look of total joy on his face.

The paragraph underneath the picture says:

One day a little boy carrying a bag of blood asked me why the people in my country never smile. I didn't know what to answer. While he looked at the blood he was carrying as a treasure to eat, he explained to me "I smile all the time, I'm lucky. Today I'm going to eat this and tomorrow I will see the sun again."

If this kid can see himself as lucky, then my *problems* are a total embarrassment. Because compared to the people of Anlong Pi, I have hit the lottery.

You see, they have no choices. They can't choose what they eat, they just eat what they find. They can't go into a shop and buy a chocolate bar if they feel like one. I used to complain that chocolate was too hard to resist. I used to say it was the chocolate company's fault for making it addictive.

But I forgot one thing. I have a choice. I chose to eat the chocolate. The people of Anlong Pi don't have the freedom to choose their food. The people of Anlong Pi live in conditions we can't even imagine, yet they are so happy. They see themselves as lucky.

You're not a victim of pregnancy

Sympathy doesn't exist beyond what people see in themselves.

I used to be a sympathy addict. When I was a fat girl, I'd whore myself out for a little taste of that emotional heroin. It's embarrassing to think that about the subtle things I'd do just so I'd be seen as a victim of something, rather than not.

I'll give you an example. This is really embarrassing to admit, but I've got to do it, to purge it from my system and should you be the same as me, give you the chance to purge it from yours.

I went to Sydney for a TV interview, where the station paid for me to be picked up by a limo and driven to my hotel that I would stay in for the night before being picked up in the morning, driven to the studio, made up, hair done and then interviewed.

This is my jam. I *love* being in front of the cameras. I'm a girl, so I *love* being treated like a princess. Make up done, hair done for me, surrounded by TV stars while I chat to them and dream about what it would be like to be as famous as them.

But the most amazing part is that I got a room to myself, with no children for a whole night. The bed was made with fresh crisp sheets and I could go to sleep as early as I wanted. To top it off, there was no cell phone reception. I knew this, Julius knew this. There would be no contact from 5pm at night until 7am the following morning.

For a mother of 5, this is a dream. A total dream come true. I thought about poor Julius and how he had to cope with all of them on his own 10,000km away. "He'll handle it, he always does. In his calm, playful way, he'll get it all done." I said to myself, but I feel guilty.

Or do I?

The night passes uneventfully as I flick through TV channels or toss and turn in my bed. In the morning when I finally get into the studio I call Julius to check in. Instead of asking how he went with all the kids, I start a rant about how bad my night was, how the TV was boring and how the sheets were too stiff.

It was too quiet in this mountain hotel and what's the point in staying so far away from the city if you get there too late to see the view. The limo driver never spoke to me and I've got a sore stomach because the barista at the hotel made my coffee too strong.

When I finally finished my tirade, Julius replied with "I'd hate to be living in your head."

Definitely not the response I was expecting, or hoping for. After yelling at him over the phone for being so insensitive, he calmly replied, "Honey, you had an opportunity to have a full night sleep, on your own. You've had the opportunity to get up whenever you want. You're about to go on TV and share your message with the country. It sounds like you've chosen to make that a bad thing. Being a victim doesn't look good on you."

And I immediately got it. I had been given a once in a parent-time opportunity to completely relax, but I was so addicted to sympathy that I turned it into a negative experience. It's so embarrassing and I've done it so many times before.

I'm so grateful that I had time on the airplane home to think about how fortunate I was, and since then I have made a point of not only being grateful, but avoiding any chance to be a victim.

Being a victim is so easy, and for most women it is the default. We live in a society where being successful is seen as lucky and bragging, so we do whatever we can to cover it up. We will find and focus on the most trivial thing to make it seem like we're underdogs.

And I totally understand not bragging, especially to our 'tall poppy' friends, but don't for a second believe the bullshit story you're telling yourself to avoid being seen as a gloat. You *are* lucky, you *are* fortunate, your life *is* great. You're pregnant! How much better can it get!

Far too many mums feel great in pregnancy and try to cover it up by searching for the morning sickness, or the cravings or staying up all night watching TV so they can feel the tiredness everyone else complains about.

You really do have a choice. You can focus on what's bad if you want. Doing so will take the crosshairs off you, but you'll feel like shit and start to believe that you are a victim of your pregnancy. Or, you can focus on what's great about being pregnant, which will make you happy, and everybody else jealous.

Or will they?

I started this chapter by saying that sympathy only exists because people see it in themselves. There's a lot to this sentence so I'll break it down.

For starters, your husband cannot see what is going on with you and formulate an accurate response in himself. He doesn't have the mechanism to do it, so don't even bother trying to get sympathy from him. He couldn't give you sincere sympathy even if he wanted to. It's like a dog trying to sympathize with a bird who can't fly.

Just let him off the hook, he's not your punching bag. And don't worry, we'll get into him soon. I'll get my husband to explain to your husband all there is to being a partner in this journey.

Next you need to understand that bad thoughts are contagious. If you complain in your mother's group about your sore back, every other mother there is going to nod with pity and agreement. They may actually be feeling better than ever (the hormones to build a baby actually flow through you too, so you can rebuild yourself). But they don't want to gloat, so they just go along with it.

Bad thoughts are contagious, but good thoughts are too. And they're so much more fun! Everything is relative too. You have no possible chance of feeling what someone else's pain is, because your only frame of reference is your own pain.

So if you were to say, "I've heard about mums with sore backs, but mine's actually not really sore at all," chances are you'll get nods of agreement.

By being positive, you are giving other mums the permission to be positive too.

Being positive is so much better for everyone than being negative. Start the trend, it'll be contagious. Wouldn't you be rather spending time pointing out things that make you feel good, like your new glowing skin, or the brightness of your eyes or the feeling of a little kick, or how much better your sex life is with all the blood in your vagina?

I know I would, given the choice.

You know you have a choice right?

You're not the victim of pregnancy. It's not something that's happened to you. You chose it. Having a baby is the emotional equivalent of winning the lottery. There's really very little to complain about if you win the lottery. You bought the ticket hoping to win, so when you do win, don't complain about it.

It starts with joy

The people of Anlong Pi hide a very interesting secret. They don't have any diseases. They get cuts and bruises from the broken glass in the dump, but they never seem to fall ill.

Which got me wondering. If they can birth healthy children, on a diet of bin juice and maggots, how important is a nutritious diet to birthing a healthy child. Are we putting too much importance on nutrition?

We're going down a deep rabbit hole here, but to avoid the issues of differing opinions, we'll just tour the rabbit hole. Just to give you a little taste of what is beneath the painted hills.

If you want to go further, that's up to you. But it's not for this book.

Ok, so a dump dweller can produce a healthy baby, and an uncomplicated birth. But I was told that I needed to have milk. I was told that I needed to eat a balanced diet of grains, meats, vegetables and everything else because I would need the energy?

Interestingly, poor people around the world seem to breed quite well. Places with the most poverty seem to be overcrowded. Africa, India and most South Pacific Islands have wide spread poverty and soaring populations. In most of these places, babies are born in shacks or huts with no medical help. We know for sure that people living on less than $2 a day aren't buying themselves milk, meat or weetbix!

What about China, a population that eats mostly rice? They don't seem to have any problems producing healthy children. I know a lot of vegans who have healthy children. No animal products at all? That's so dangerous, right? I even know some raw food enthusiasts who have had beautiful, healthy children. No animal products and no cooking?

What about the quintessential Aussie bogan, living off a diet of fast food and soft drink, who somehow manages to have many, many healthy children?

So what do you eat for a healthy baby?

Well, here's how I see it. The baby inside you is essentially behaving like a parasite. It's making sure that it is well fed by taking what it needs from you. Whether you're living off bin juice, big mac's or broccolini, your baby will be fine. It will take what it needs from you, and no more.

Do you find it interesting that newborn babies seem to all be around the same size, no matter whether the mother is morbidly obese or underweight, rich or poor?

Your baby is selfish. It's a survivalist. You not eating *correctly* has very little impact on the little one's outcome. So whether you eat for two, or eat for you; your baby makes sure it comes first. The only person affected by your eating is going to be you.

Now don't be dramatic and start saying "this chick's crazy, she's saying my baby is a parasite and selfish." Please don't read something that's not between the lines. What I'm saying is that your baby is going to be fine. Short of getting drunk or messed up on drugs, your baby will be fine. So that piece of chocolate you're feeling so guilty about, forget it.

The guilt is far worse for your baby than the junk food.

And here's where my personal experience comes in. I was an obese mother. I was a fit mother. I've been a broke mother and a wealthy mother. But none of that mattered to my babies. They all came out similar size and healthy. The difference, was in me.

So back to the last section. It starts with Joy. You know how I said that Alexis projects my moods? Well, what if the only thing we actually give our kids is our emotion.

Fat, skinny, rich or poor, it's the stressed women who have the complicated births. Happy mums have easy births. What if the only thing you can control about being given to your baby is the emotion you feed it. Everything else is filtered by the placenta. Emotion doesn't pass through the blood. It's felt. You don't even have to be in the same country as someone to be affected by their emotions.

I share the emotion with characters in movies. If they cry, I cry. I'm sure you're the same. Emotions aren't carried in the wind, they can jump time and space. So what is the number one purpose for a pregnant mum?

Joy.

Think about it like this. When someone has their first baby, they suddenly find so much joy in their lives. Now think how emotionally exhausting it is to convince your friend Debbie Downer that life is actually pretty good. How tired are you just earning a smile off her?

Imagine how hard your baby is working to give you joy. It's meant to be spending all it's energy growing. But it has to make you happy. Now, imagine if you could just be happy. If you didn't rely on your baby to make you happy. What sort of unhindered life could your baby have now?

Take it a step further, what if you gave your baby joy? We've now gone from hindering a baby, to unhindering it, to giving it a boost in this game called life.

Can you see what I'm getting at?

Being happy isn't enough. You've got to project it. Your baby needs to feel it from you, so that it can have the boosted start in life I know you want to give it.

Emotional Imprinting

So how do you do it?

Well, it starts with you realizing that you are not the victim of pregnancy. You've been blessed. You've been chosen out of all the women on earth to bring a new soul into the world.

You are solely responsible for the wellbeing of this soul. I like to imagine life as a holiday, I've got 5 little holiday makers in my care, and I'm their chaperone. Do I give them a good experience, show them all that is great and exciting and fun about this holiday destination?

I never used to think like this. I used to take pregnancy for granted. Quickly the gift of birth loses it's gloss in the afterglow. Nappies and cracked nipples mixed with sleepless nights bear down on the spirit like a ton of bricks.

But I don't live on a dump. I may not have much sleep, but I have a bed. I have a home. I have a healthy child who is engaging with me, relying on me to give it experiences. It's trusting me to give it whatever I choose. Bad experiences or good ones, it doesn't make requests. It doesn't judge. It just exists, moment to moment, in a state of excited interest.

Whether you bring a baby up on a dump site or a palace, the only thing you can control is their emotional connection and experience with this world. And that comes directly from you to start with.

As the baby grows, it will be subjected to other influential emotional hosts. Like brothers, sisters, dad, teachers etc. But for the first 9 months, it can only get it's emotional imprint from you. It's mother.

For food and drink, it relies on your placenta. Yes, that food and drink still has to be eaten by you, but the placenta *filters* it. For emotions, it relies directly on you.

And here's the conundrum. Your emotions rely heavily on your experience of your environment. You have 2 of them. External, and internal. Whether you are happy with your life as it currently is, plays a huge role in the happiness of your child. But just as importantly what you eat, what environment you expose your insides to, plays a huge part in your babies eventual wellbeing.

You can change your attitude to your external environment, and let's face it, a lot of us don't have much choice in the environment. We do have a choice as to how we process that environment and our attitudes toward it. So start by being content that where you are right now, is where you are meant to be. If you get a strong gut feel that it's not right, then you need to change it to something that makes you feel content in your gut.

But the catch here is to not do anything for anyone else. Don't move into a bigger house or a different neighbourhood because your friend has more monety than you and you want to keep up. To give you an example, we actually moved to a smaller house because we had strong gut feels that we were spending too much on the big fancy house. And we were right.

Back to your internal environment. What's easier? Change your attitude towards your food, or change your food?

Interesting question, right?

Let's say you're eating junk food and you don't like that you are. Is it easier to convince yourself that you should be OK with junk food, or is it just easier to eat something that feels right?

Of course eating something that feels right is easier. I've done it. I don't like that I'm eating dairy, and no matter how I justified it to myself, I had this deep gut feeling that I was doing something that didn't agree with me. I tried to convince myself my whole life that I needed dairy.

One day I decided to get rid of that feeling of unease by just eating something different. Something that I liked. I like nuts, so I made milk out of nuts. When I eat something with nut milk, I can feel an internal emotional response. My body makes me feel good, and in turn I feel good. Feeling good about what you put inside you dictates half of your emotion. The other half comes from your external environment.

Sometimes it's very hard to change the external environment. But the internal environment can be changed in one meal. Try it. Eat something that you *know* your body will love you for, and see how much happier you are.

Just sit quietly for a few minutes and *feel* what you might want to eat. Is it a punnet of blueberries? A quinoa salad? If you ignore the addictive eating (junk foods) you'll find what your body loves. When you find it, eat it.

You see, the body is resourceful, but it's like a blind guy at a buffet. It will take anything, hoping to find something it likes. So it tells you to just keep feeding it. What you'll find is that once you listen to your body, and eat for joy… hunger dissipates.

That longing for some chocolate disappears. Because your body is getting what it wants. Love. Chocolate makes you feel like you're being loved chemically, but if you're actually loving yourself; you won't need the cheap chemical counterpart.

And what makes this even more interesting is when you add love from your partner. If you become happier, by changing your internal environment, you'll want an outlet for your joy. You'll give it to him, and in turn; he'll give it back to you. So not only are you improving your internal environment by loving it, you're improving your external environment by loving your partner, who will love you back.

Before long, the cascading effect of it will evolve into a cataclysmic experience of pure joy. Like an orgasm that just never ends. You can live in that moment forever. And if that's not a good enough example, or a long time ago, just imagine being able to eat chocolate without guilt. What you're really wanting is to feel *in love* without the deep feeling that you're doing it *the wrong way*.

Chemical happiness (chocolate) can never replace internal, projected happiness. Bi-angle, internal and external experience of joy that lasts forever and gets stronger the more you feel it will make chocolate love seem like a crayon drawing.

You deserve to be the happiest person on earth. You, the baby you carry and everyone else in your immediate influence deserves to see your happiness. And best of all, the more you love, the more you receive.

And it all starts from inside. Internal environment. What you eat.

Purpose and Ambition

If there's one thing you can get out of this book, it's that you need to be happy. If you can master that, you're going to live the most empowering life as a mother. You and your children will benefit from it in ways that are simply inexplicable.

And yeah, it sounds cheesy and one of those "yeah, righto" kindo of things, but being happy is actually not that hard. You see, we humans put so much pressure on ourselves.

Expectations? Nobody knows what's coming up for you in your life, so why put expectations on yourself. I know, I'm starting to sound like a martyr because I appear to have huge expectations on myself. But I can tell you I'm not doing things that I don't feel from inside.

There is a difference between purposeful movement and ambition. I have learnt to calm my head voice, the one that says "why does that girl deserve to have that car…" or "it's not fair that you are shorter than her." And it may seem trivial and ditsy, but it's true, everyone has that voice. I've learnt to quiet it, and listen to the purpose driver.

And here's how I know what my driver is. Ever since I can remember, I've had this drive to help people be better. As a young girl, I thought I was going to get there through TV. I couldn't get into TV, so I settled into a career in radio. But I never got a proper gig, or too entrenched in the success of radio.

For nearly 10 years I was in radio, and on the side was keeping fit and experimenting with my nutrition. I thought that's what other people did. I thought that's what other people enjoyed doing in their spare time. Exercise and nutrition were what my mind drifted to. People would naturally gravitate to me and ask me fitness questions, or food questions.

All of these things were signs. I didn't know it then, but they certainly were. Then one day out of the blue, I was doing a live cross at a personal training academy close to home and the owner just so happened to be there at the same time.

Somehow, and I really don't know how, I started my personal training course the next week, on a full scholarship. I had quit my 10 year career on a whim, with no chance of returning. But it felt right.

I've never looked back. I've never looked back. Until now, as I reminisce for you at the interesting turns of fate in my life. Don't get me wrong though, there have been many, many times that I've wondered if I was on the right path.

But I know I am because even if I think about another career, I seem to drift back to fitness. And that's where I want you to spend a bit of time thinking about what it is that you have always dreamed about. What it is that drives you. What you find easy, what you make your hobby.

See there's a difference between purpose and ambition. They feel very similar, but there is a difference. To me, purpose feels like this: "When I die and look back on my life, will I be content?"

Purpose is not material. Ambition is. Ambition is that feeling you get when you test drive a sports car. It can be far more powerful than purpose, but ambition fades. If I think back to all the cars, handbags, shoes and other material things that have given me that rise in energy; I can't think of one that has lasted longer than a few months.

Being a mum and in particular being pregnant has a little trap that you want to be aware of. It may not seem it, but parenting is fraught with ambition. "I want the best pram, I'm going to have the home birth, or the private hospital suite. I'm going to have a push ring, I'm going to have the best baby announcement picture." All of these things are ambitions. And they're not a bad thing, just try not to get too caught up in them, because in the end nobody cares.

I've done it and I've seen it too many times to count. I wanted to look like a rich mum in an Audi Q7. Thank god I couldn't afford one, because the inside of our van is trashed. 5 kids, and we've allowed them to eat in the car. We've got our own version of the Anlong Pi dump.

And the coolest thing is nobody gives a shit. Nobody cares if we have this Hyundai iMax or the Q7, because in the end everybody seems to only be thinking about themselves and their own ambitions anyway. Try to avoid getting caught up in your ambitions. Because beneath them, like a constantly flowing river, is your purpose.

You now have an excuse

So what's the point.

Well, you have now got an excuse. Pregnancy is one of those times in your life that you can make sudden, drastic changes and it's not only understandable, but expected.

Imagine your husband telling his boss that he needs time off "to find himself." He'll probably get laughed out of his job. But if you're pregnant, your boss will *expect* you to do it. It's milestones in life like this that bring you alongside your purpose. Everyone else knows it or can feel it.

So use this time to find your purpose. Find out what makes you happy and *go do it*!

You have an excuse. People use this opportunity to do really bad things to themselves, like get fat as hell or buy every baby carrier ever invented. You can seriously do the weirdest shit and people will make the excuse for you.

If you've been afraid of battling with your mother in law, even though you have that burning gut feel that you need to say something, now's the time. Give her an earful. Tear her a new arse. She'll understand. She'll probably be very proud of you. She's been there before, with her own mother in law.

That's a really negative example, but one most of us can relate to. If you've always felt a drive to paint, or work with animals, or do yoga all day, now is your chance to do it. Do you love food and dream of having your own food blog – ... DO...IT!

Because if you've been dreaming about it for a long time, and you've always had an excuse for why you can't, now's your chance. It may be the last chance you ever get. And when you get to the end of your life, will you look back and regret it?

You'll regret it if you said no, and then look back at what you actually did. You actually spend the time worrying about ambitions and expectations. Instead of going with the flow of your purpose.

And how do you know you're on purpose? It's simple. You'll feel unbridled joy while you do it. Joy that seeps through to the rest of your life. You see, the only thing stopping you from doing what you are meant to do, instead of what you think you should do, is you. Your ambition.

"I can't start a yoga studio, I'm a lawyer." Is something you never want to say, because you are sacrificing your purpose for money. And if you are living in your purpose, money is ineffectual.

Right now, you may be stressing about money all the time. But as soon as you start doing what you love, what makes you happy, money no longer becomes an instrument of joy. Just like chocolate no longer becomes your substitute for love.

I've been pretty firm about finding your purpose and pursuing it, and I need to be, because once the baby is out, and you're a full time mother, you won't have the same amount of time it takes to dive into your purpose.

But this chapter is about finding joy. Joy doesn't just come from living your purpose. It's certainly a big part of it, but it's not the only string in your happiness violin. We touched on food before and we'll revisit it now.

Eat what makes you shine. Take your time choosing your food. Take your time choosing your actions. You don't need to make snap decisions. In fact, you can take as long as you want to make decisions.

Have you ever wondered why you feel like you need to make decisions so fast? Maybe it was because of school exams. But that exam mindset is never going to serve you in your quest for happiness. Stressing about a decision doesn't allow you to dive into your purpose. You will always be guided by ambition if you're stressed.

You need to learn to slow down. Slow down. Take time. I like to say diving into your purpose, because to me that's what it feels like. If I'm feeling hungry, I'll sit in silence for a few minutes and dive through the ambitious decisions (like fast food) and wait to see what my body tells me I really want.

This sounds all woo woo and hippy, but it's not. It's sensible and it's logical. If people just thought about what their bodies really wanted to eat, they'd never stop at a drive through take away. We all know that fast food is bad for us, so if you decide based on what will make you happy, then you'll remember that about 20 minutes after eating fast food, you feel terrible. Guilty, sick and worst of all, still hungry, because you didn't eat what your body wanted, so it's still asking you for it.

It's the difference between a distracted life and a focused life. Focused people are so much calmer. Distracted people are always fidgeting, stressing, getting things wrong, spending money, eating mindlessly.

People tell me that they don't have to time to dive into their purpose for every decision. But that's a lie. I used to believe it, and I used to lie to myself about it. But my phone disagrees.

Think about how much time you spend scrolling through your phone. All that time could be used to calm your thoughts and dive into your purpose. And the more you do it, the easier it gets, and the faster you get at doing it. You'll learn to recognize when you are making decisions without it, and you'll recognize when you are.

You'll feel more sure. For example, you'll take a moment to decide on what to eat, and then you won't change your mind. Distracted thinking is when you decide, then change your mind, then change it back and then just go to the closest place.

Think about this chapter for a little while. It's not meant to be a sermon, but if you don't get it, then I'm afraid you're just not ready for it. Just not ready to be happy, your ambition is standing in the way, so firmly planted that you think it's you.

But if you're unhappy in your life. Any part of it, then you are a victim of your own expectations and ambitions. Learn to recognize them for what they are and ignore them. Take a moment to dive deep into your purpose and you'll be amazed at how easy it is to stay happy, upbeat and positive.

Even in the most trying external circumstances.

How to dive into your purpose

There's a lady I know called Avril. Deep wrinkles criss-cross her face and her eyes shine with depth of sorrow only her god can understand. In the grooves of her face lie stories untold.

Avril doesn't speak. But she has a presence that can be felt. Avril is not mute, she chooses not to speak. I don't know why, she's never told me (on account of the fact that she doesn't speak). But I don't actually want to know why.

I don't want to know in case it is something simple. Like she can't speak English.

I like to believe that she doesn't speak, because she prefers to listen. She prefers to listen so much that she chooses not to speak. Under the leathery exterior is a soul, journeyed here from who knows where, leaving soon, but nobody knows when.

Deep beneath the wrinkles is a soul who gets it. She doesn't need to speak, because every time she speaks, she's not listening. The answers are not in what you say. The answers are not found in discussion or opinion.

The answers to everything in your life are within you. Under the makeup, under the skin, behind the eyes. They say that the eyes are the window to the soul. When I sit in front of Avril, I run out of trivial things to say and just end up looking at her. She looks back. Always looking at me.

At first it's kind of funny, then confronting, then when I think about giving up, the magic happens. A calmness descends around us, or from her. We're connected. Not in an electric way, but in a way that makes us feel like we're sharing a journey. I look into Avril's eyes and I see myself. I see *all* of myself.

And I instantly become content. Focused but content. In the headlights of her stare, I see every lie I've ever told. Every regret I've ever had. I feel honest. And I feel OK about it. I feel like, in the safety of her silent stare, I am where I am meant to be.

I don't know about her. Staring into my face, she sometimes weeps. Sometimes laughs. Mostly, she just looks like she's staring into a desolate wilderness. Avril has so much sadness. So much sadness.

I don't know why she's so sad. I don't want to know. It's got nothing to do with me, if she one days breaks her silence and shares her stories with me, It will become my business, but in the meantime I use her, the way she uses me. To get clarity. To get understanding. To dive into purpose. To come close to the very fabric of our existence.

When I stare into Avril's eyes, I see things I could never see on my own. It's my version of meditation.

I've known Avril for over a decade. Each time I visit her, it's the same. I ask her carers how she is and they give a terse response. "Cranky," or "good today." I never ask any more, because Avril has *always* been with me. I feel like I known her for many, many lifetimes.

I met Avril years ago, sitting on the train home from Brisbane. She was staring at me from across the carriage with a cheeky grin. As soon as I had the courage to look back, I felt the magnetism. I felt the power in her stare.

I was tired and just, completely out of character, decided to stare back at her. At first, I thought she was blind, or looking past me. But we were close and I could see into her eyes. I could see she was staring into mine. Never looking anywhere else, just into my eyes.

By the time I got to my stop, I felt like the weight of the world had lifted from my shoulders. I began to speak to her and she immediately turned away. At the time I didn't think anything of it, but I now know that this must be what the carers at her nursing home must mean when they say she's "cranky."

A few weeks later, I saw her again. Running past a bus stop, I noticed her standing there. Like hitting a brick wall, I stopped. She was looking back at me with that calm, cheeky half smile. I muttered something and she just turned away.

For months I kept running into her. At the supermarket. At the library. She even turned up to one of my speaking events, sat in the background and left before I got the chance to thank her.

"She seems to light up when she sees you" said her carer one day at Woolworths. You should come around and visit her some time. She's not one for speaking, but if you have the time, we'd really love to see her smile like that more often.

Before I knew it, I was visiting this quirky old lady once, maybe twice a week. I never felt compelled to speak. I just sat there and looked around the room, at the other people and eventually at her.

Like a magnet clicking, I'd be drawn into her stare. The half smile would return and for an unimaginable time, we'd be locked in this apparent stare off. After a few years, people just thought I was related to her. A granddaughter. She's never had another visitor that I know of, just me.

I don't get to see her much anymore on account of my tribe of kids, but when I somehow find the time, I feel like I've needed it. Deep in those eyes lie the secrets of my life. The answers to my unanswerable questions.

But that's not all. I look into her eyes and I see myself. All of myself. Naked and innocent like a newborn baby. I long ago tried it with Julius and found it to be the same. We've never spoken to anyone else about it until Josh came home from acting school saying that he'd done an exercise where he had to stare into someone else's eyes for over an hour. He described the same enlightening experience.

Somehow, staring into someone else's eyes we get to see the truth of our lives. If you struggle with diving into your purpose, try it. Find someone, a friend or your husband and book an hour where you just stare into one another's eyes.

I'd go so far as to say, before your baby is born, please look into your husband's eyes. You and he will see each other as you first met. You will fall in love again. Deeper than before. Then, after you've secured that love, his eyes will become mirrors. You'll drift to yourself. You'll touch your purpose, so dive deep into it and enjoy the experience.

Deep in the eyes of your husband, you'll see what you're meant to do with your life. You'll be content and focused. But most important of all... You'll be happy again.

Do that, then immediately upon waking, decide what you want to eat. After this exercise, decisions of purpose will dominate decisions of ego, or ambition. Do it as often or as little as you like. But just promise yourself you'll do it once.

Pretty soon you'll have a little baby to feed. Feeding babies stare the same way Avril does. They stare with unfaltering love at you. When you stare back into their deep azure eyes, you'll see more than just yourself. You'll see the purpose and design of the entire universe.

Joyful eating

To find out what you should eat, I find it easier to talk about what you shouldn't eat. Because it's a lot smaller list than what you *should* eat.

Think about it like this. Your child is going to be an adult one day, and they will ask you, "what should I do with my life?"

What a powerful question. A chance for a mother to truly add value to her child's life. Old school mums would say, "find a rich man." Our mums would probably say something based on what we're good at, like "you should be a lawyer, because you're very convincing" or "you're good with your hands, so do a trade."

That's a good start, and it very well may be the right answer, but what if it isn't? What if you always wanted to be a ballerina, or tank driver. What if you were destined to be a musician as influential as lady gaga, and you ended up being a nurse, because you didn't mind the sight of blood?

So us new age mums would not even give a suggestion. We'd say, "Do whatever makes you truly happy."

But that's such a wishy washy answer when it comes to food, because there are different levels of happy, as we've discussed before. So I find it works well to then clarify by listing things that you probably shouldn't do with your life (or shouldn't eat).

"As long as you don't commit crimes, do whatever it is that makes you happy"

That eliminates becoming a murderer, a drug dealer, a lawyer and any other bad career choice. Don't sue me for that joke, I know some really lovely drug dealers.

They're called pharmacists.

I'm just messing with you now.

So when it comes to food, I would say "eat anything that makes you truly happy, as long as it's not bad for you."

And use logic when it comes to what's bad for you. The latest diet trend is not logic, unless it makes sense to you. Don't follow fads, make up your own mind. You'll know what's wrong because you'll feel like shit after you've eaten it. You'll know what's right because you'll feel wonderful after eating it. You'll feel better than before you ate it.

It really is that simple. Just have a private conversation with yourself. Like this:

Do you ever feel vibrant and better after eating fast food?

No.

Well then, fast food is bad for you.

Do you ever feel vibrant and better after drinking a green juice?

Yes, I feel lighter and cleaner.

So green juice is good for you. Apple juice?

Tastes good.

What about after say 5mins-30 mins?

I get a sore gut and dry mouth. I feel hungry.

Does that make you feel better than before you drank it?

No.

Apple Juice is off the menu.

What if I try juicing apples.

Sure, do you feel better after having them?

No. I feel more tired.

Right, even juiced apples are off. What if you try eating the apple?

Granny Smith's are in season, I'll try one.

[later] how was it?

Really good. I felt more energetic for about 2 hours afterwards. My mouth felt cleaner and my stomach felt satisfied.

Would you say you benefited from eating it?

Yes.

Green apples can stay on the menu.

See how easy that is? Seriously that's all there is to it. You and your inside voice, having a creepy little private conversation about food. You do talk to yourself, don't you?

Just me?

Start with a list of things you know you don't like. Then a list of things you like to eat, but you know don't serve you well. Then a list of things you're unsure of. You'll be left with a pretty big list of things you can eat.

So just eat them!

Nutrition vs Energy

Fat, proteins and carbs. You hear about these all the time. The low fat diet. The low carb diet. The high protein diet.

Here's the scoop.

Fats and carbs are energy sources. They provide you with energy to do what you need to do for the day. Just like your car. Carbs are like petrol. They allow the car to run, they power the car. But there is another fuel on board a car. It's the battery. In the human, the battery isn't just a small 12V square thing under the hood. Its your fat stores.

In a car, the battery charges until it's full. In a human, the battery has no 'full'. It will keep on charging as long as you keep on pumping more energy into it.

The more you put into it, the more it stores, it's only requirement is space. The more energy you add into your battery, the more space it requires to store it, so it just gets bigger.

Eventually it gets so big that you begin to feel it. You feel heavier. And just like a car, the heavier you are, the more energy you're going to need to get going every day *and* the more problems you're going to have. If you start loading a Hyundai Getz with the load a truck is meant to carry, it won't last long before it breaks down.

Same with a human. And just like a car, when a human gets too heavy, it becomes almost too hard to move around like it used to, so we do things differently, we try not to use the car unless it's absolutely necessary. That's OK if it's a car, but when a human sits in the garage doing nothing, it's compelled to do one thing. Eat.

Now here's an interesting insight. One kilogram of fat contains 9,000 calories. An average sized woman needs only 1500 calories per day to survive. So that means, for every excess kilo of fat you're carrying, you can survive for 6 days *without eating a damn thing*.

If you have 10 kilos to lose, you can mathematically survive 60 days without eating anything.

But before you go starving yourself and your baby, you need to understand this. Calories are just energy. You would probably die well before then, because you'd be missing something so much more important than energy in. You'd be missing *nutrition*.

There is a very, very big difference between energy and nutrition. Proteins are nutrition, because they are used for more than just energy. Vitamins, minerals, antioxidants, amino acids, peptides, and many many other things are required to keep a body from succumbing to the environment we live in.

Even more interesting is that your body almost *never* pesters you for energy. The hunger you feel is actually for nutrition. We've unfortunately, through the miracles of food science and the pressures of money, been brought up in a world where we believe that hunger means *more energy*.

Imagine if every time the oil light came on in your car, you just went to the petrol station and filled up on fuel. About 10 minutes after you left the fuel station, the light would come back on. So you went back and filled up on fuel again. Eating for energy is *just like that*!

Unless you are extremely lean, your body has enough energy on board to run itself. Remember, for every kilo of fat, you can survive for 6 days.

Even me at my leanest – let's say at 58kg I am 12% body fat. That's 7 kilos of body fat I can use up. 7x6 is 6 weeks before I've completely exhausted my fuel supply.

So, why do we feel hungry? It's for things that are far more important. Nutrition. Building blocks. A human body is always regenerating itself. And while you're growing a baby inside you, you're regenerating yourself *and your baby*.

It takes energy to do it, so you have a higher energy need, but - and this is a big *BUT* - our body and your baby's body can't be built on fuel alone. That's like building a car out of petrol.

A car is built to last 20 years or so. A human body is built to last at most a couple of hours before a part dies and needs to be replaced by a new one. Think about the complexity of a human body. Cars don't have to think, they don't have emotions, they don't breed, they don't have to *go to work*, they don't grow, they don't talk. Our bodies perform so many complex tasks, and we're made out of cells, not steel. Cells die. It's like building a moving hotel out of grass clippings.

Isn't the human body amazing! Think about it for a minute, all the things we're able to do, and all the things you've done, in a body that spends all day rebuilding itself. But most people think all we need is more energy.

Hell no! If you keep pumping more energy in than your body needs, it's going to use up some of the resources required to keep it safe from harm, to store that energy. I don't know about you, but I want my body to be fully focussed on *now*. On the baby growing in my stomach. Not distracted by finding a place to stash the excess fuel I keep shovelling into my mouth.

Worse still, if you're only eating for energy, chances are you're eating something designed to give you lots more energy per bite. Like a cheeseburger. Eating a cheeseburger because you're hungry is like pulling into a service station for air in your tyres and leaving with a fuel tanker on your roof racks.

Cheeseburgers and any other processed food for that matter, have been stripped of any useable nutrition, and are essentially energy bombs! Not only that, they're prevented from falling apart or being edible by any other living organism, by the same chemicals used to kill cockroaches. And you know how hard it is to kill a cockroach!

The manufacturer calls it a *preservative*, but I call it a congenital defect. Numbers aren't food. Food is food. Food is nutrition, and lucky for us, it comes packaged with energy!

How exciting is that! If you eat for nutrition, you'll get the energy as a bonus. If you eat for energy, you'll get no nutrition.

Eating for nutrition is actually much easier than eating for energy! Nature has made it so easy, even a child can do it. Nature has been so kind to us dumb humans that it's even colour coded nutrition for us so we can recognise it!

Fruits, vegetables, nuts and seeds all have different colours. Each colour represents a very important nutritional component needed by your body. Reds, greens, oranges, yellows, blues, purples, browns, blacks, whites and every shade in between.

How cool is that, why would nature, or God or the Universe ever make it colour coded, surely it would be much easier to make all food a single colour? Most animals only eat food of one colour. Grass is green. Cows only eat grass. But a cow is not a human, humans are capable of much more... So, so much more.

Can you believe though, that a cow can do all the things a cow can do, simply by eating grass. In fact most animals on earth survive off only greens. There's a clue there! Most of what we need to survive is in the colour green. How much green food are you eating at the moment. Does it make up 90% of your daily diet? 95%?

Because really, greens should be the backbone of your diet. Greens. Leaves. Lettuce leaves. Spinach leaves etc.

We're more complicated than the cow, so we need a bit more than that, but you know what, it's not much! Just a few more colours. About 5% of our diets needs to be made up of a few more colours. That's it!

That is until you pollute your body. Live in a city, and you need to have more colours. Just to combat the pollution. Add some stress and you'll need to have more colours, just to protect you from yourself. Add some chemicals from the nutrition bombs you've been eating and you're going to need more colours!

Is it starting to come together for you?

Can you see how the most important step is to Just. Be. Happy?

Cows are happy, so all they need to eat is grass. If you were deeply happy, all you'd need to eat was greens. Expectations and ambitions are like junk food. They add stress to your body and you have to combat that.

It's the chicken and the egg. Be happy, and all you'll need to eat are greens. Eat mostly greens, and you'll begin to feel happy!

Draw your own rainbow

Greens carry with them an enormous amount of nutrition, as well as a little bit of energy. More than enough energy to keep us alive for many many years. But you haven't been living in a tropical paradise, feasting on only greens and living a life of pure bliss have you?

So, like me, you'll need to add in some colour. You've probably heard the saying that you need to eat a rainbow of colour, but that means equal amounts of each colour. I like to look at the whole picture. A rainbow doesn't appear on it's own. It's usually over a lush meadow of green and in a sky of blue. At least in children's paintings – remember that nature designed nutrition to be easy for kids to understand.

So eat as much green as the meadow in the picture. Drink as much water as the sky is blue, and top yourself up with a rainbow of happiness!

But what about meat?

Meat is like religion. Some people swear it's important, others swear it is what's wrong with the world. I'm going to stand on the fence and say that in my picture of the rainbow in the sky, there happens to be a cow in the meadow. It certainly doesn't take up the entire picture, but it's there because I like it. To me, it feels incomplete without it.

Some days, however, my picture has no cow. It may have a chicken. Or a sheep. Or nothing. Many people don't put animals in their pictures and interestingly, they don't die.

Many vegans or vegetarians are healthier than people who eat meat, but that's not because meat is bad for you, it's because most people who eat meat, have rainbow picture that looks like used toilet paper. It's all streaky browns and whites. Maybe a tiny token piece of green, but certainly not a meadow!

So, whether you eat meat or not, you still have to make the meadow in your rainbow picture the biggest part. And don't go judging other people's art. If they can't be bothered painting it and instead take a big shit on the paper, by all means help them get some life perspective. But if you've got it mostly right and you have a seagull in your picture, who am I to judge?

Unless it's neon.

The colour green should be a natural colour green. Not an overly bright colour green. Same with the rainbow. Don't be fooled by some cash hungry profiteering imposter who trys to sell you paint that will make your picture so much brighter than the real thing. Be a realist, not an impressionist or a cartoon artist. Try and match the real thing.

Fake colours are like preservatives, they don't even have real names, they have numbers.

Draw a rainbow in a clear blue sky, above a large green meadow and you'll never need to know anything else about food.

And that about sums up nutrition.

Why exercise?

Which means we'll move right into exercise, and I'll start with the biggest misconception about exercise there is: Exercise makes you lose weight.

Exercise does not make you lose weight. My husband gained weight while training for an ultra-marathon. He ran over 100km every week. That's more than 10 hours of the hardest cardiovascular exercise. He also did weights 5 days a week and competed in crossfit tournaments to increase his VO_2max.

Well, he increased his VO_2max, but concurrently increased his waist size. Because the man that I married has an appetite that would compete with a boys' boarding school, and when training, his body screamed for food.

We didn't know the difference between nutrition and energy at the time, so he just opened the throttle on his eating. He thought, "I'm training this much, I'll need a lot of food." And he wasn't eating junk food. Oats and pasta formed the bulk of his diet, but even that was enough to make him fatten up.

Contrast that with many, many people who just diet. The weight just seems to fall off them with little or no effort.

Which begs the question; why exercise?

If you don't exercise for weight loss, why do so many people have gym memberships. Why do so many people go running or cycling? We've always been told that to lose weight we need to exercise, right?

Exercise does not make you lose weight for two reasons. Firstly, if you exercise for weight loss, you tend to over exercise. Like Julius did. Overexercising stresses the body, which responds by nagging you for more nutrition. Which is felt as hunger. So you eat more. More than you burnt in fact, because a 10km run doesn't even burn enough energy to justify a Big Mac.

So for most people, exercise to diet means an increase in food. Combine that with the old "I exercised for 45 minutes, I *deserve* an icecream tonight" attitude and you can see why gyms are crowded with overweight fit people. Never after dinner though, too full from the icecream, right?

The second reason people shouldn't use exercise to lose weight is that the exercise done is rarely enough to stimulate a metabolic response big enough. Combined with the overcompensative eating we just discussed – most 'exercise to lose weight' people just can't seem to lose weight, much to their frustration.

Which is what we want to avoid. Once again, stress – be it physical or emotional – is something we want to avoid as much as possible. Exercising to lose weight puts your body under stress, but the slow weight loss puts your mind under stress. Stress stops the release of a hormone called cortisol. Cortisol regulates the availability of fat from your body to be used as fuel.

The more stressed you are, the less fat your body allows you to use – it's like it locks up the fat. So you feel hungry. Not only for nutrition, but for calories. Your body is not giving them to you, because it's spending too much time dealing with stress. "So you better get some food into me," it says. "And make it easy, I don't want to have to cook or clean."

Recognise this behaviour?

It gets worse. Because easy food usually contains high levels of fat and sugar. Sugar raises blood insulin, which makes you feel tired. For stress, it's a coping mechanism. Avoid stress by falling asleep. But who on earth can just go to sleep whenever they want? So we eat more *energy food*. Cycle repeat.

You're lucky, because you can't exercise to lose weight while you're pregnant, so the excuse has been made for you.

On a side note, if you *are* stressed, the best thing for you is to go to sleep. When I was losing weight and I could feel the addicitve foods pulling at me, making me stressed and angry, I'd have 3 options.

1. Eat the junk and be fat. Which would make me angry the next day.
2. Storm around the house angry and destroy relationships, which would make me feel even more like eating junk. Which I'd eventually do, and then be angry the next day
3. Go to sleep. Don't eat the junk. Have nice dreams. Feel better about myself in the morning.

But that only works at night.

So what can we do?

Well, there is a 4th option. You could always exercise for *fun*.

Hating exercise will make you stressed. Stress will make you unhappy. Unhappy people get fat easier than happy people. The most critical ingredient for health is happiness.

If you do something you hate, you'll not be happy. Duh. But if you do something you hate, to lose weight? You'll become one of these women who tried every diet and every gym and can point out something wrong with all of them.

If you hate exercise, don't do it. You're better off not doing any exercise at all. Just like the people who only diet to lose weight.

But.

Of course there's a *but*.

Exercise can be one of the easiest, cheapest and most effective ways to make you happy. Happy people are healthy people. Happiness is addictive, just like being a sad sack of complaints is addictive.

I know what I'd rather be addicted to. I bet you've never enjoyed being Debbie Downer all the time. I used to go to sleep thinking that everyone in the world was *just so damn annoying!*

Great attitude that was. It certainly served me well. I pushed away all my closest friends, alienated my husband and argued with every person I came in contact with. But everybody was just so damn annoying…

To me. Which was the only thing every annoying person had in common. Me.

So I chose to be happy. And it's just that easy.

I did things to make me happy. If it didn't make me happy, I stopped. I stopped going to the gym, because it made me feel like shit. I was fat, angry and felt judged (which by the way is how everybody in every gym feels).

But I quit exercising.

At about the same time, Julius quit exercising for a purpose too. Instead of spending most of the night running, he wanted to spend time with me. He liked the new me, the not-so-highly-strung me.

He started to lose weight. So did I. By doing things to make me happy, I had decided to eat mostly greens. Quite by accident or trial and error, I felt it made me an overall happier person.

Julius just wanted me to be happy, so he ate the same as me.

After a few weeks of not exercising, we felt so good that we just went for a walk. He told me my legs looked nice and I liked the shape of his leaner calves. We held hands. He playfully smacked me on my bum and ran off. I chased him. Before you know it we were playing tag like little kids.

Weeks of inactivity meant we were quite unfit, so after about 15 minutes, we were laying on the ground puffed. But we both felt *amazing!*

It was then that I decided two things. Exercise for me would always be about happiness. I had forgotten about the joy of exercise. Somehow when I left school, exercise went from fun (sport) to a chore (gym). Not any more. I would only ever do exercise that made me feel joy.

The second thing I decided was that I wouldn't restrict myself to a time. I wouldn't exercise for *at least an hour* any more. I would just exercise until I felt like I wasn't enjoying it any more.

And the results were amazing. Exercise to me is like having sex. Sometimes it's good when it goes for long, sometimes it's good when it goes for a really short intense few minutes. But you never say to your husband "I'm going to do doggie style for 15 minutes, have a rest, then do 3 sets of cowgirl and finish with a warm down of missionary. That should be the 45 minutes for the day." Imagine how shit your sex life would be.

I bet if your husband read that he'd beg to differ!!

But you get what I mean, right? Exercise should be spontaneous and done for pleasure. For fun. Do that, and it will never be a chore. Do it well, and your body will respond. That hormone I was telling you about before, cortisol – it has a friend called serotonin. It's like the ying for it's yang. It's the feel good drug – it's the one that makes your body open the doors to the fat cells. It's the one that allows full access to your fat, making you feel not hungry.

Remember how little sleep and how little food you could survive on when you first fell deeply in love?

That's the serotonin. Fall in love with yourself again. Do exercise that makes you happy, gives you pleasure. Makes you feel in love. Hell, make love to your husband as much as you feel like it – as long as it's fun and enjoyable and gives you pleasure – 5 minutes of a passionate quickie in the kitchen is better than an hour at the gym, hating every minute!

Sex is a great exercise. And if you're at home by yourself starting to feel stressed and you can't go to sleep, why not get your vibrator out and drain a pack of batteries. Buzz yourself to happiness. I know when I have a great orgasm (or two or three) I don't feel like eating junk. I feel sexy and vibrant and I want to exercise or eat something nutritious and green and good for me. I'm sure whenever you have great sex you feel positive and happy and vibrant. Everyone around you seems *just so friendly and nice!*

Exercise and sexercise are two things you can do to make you happy. Happy people are healthy people. Happiness is addictive and it makes you a better person. Happy people are attractive and their happiness is contagious.

Be happy. Be sexy. Be you. You are sexy. You may feel like you're swelling and getting heavy and gross, but nothing can be sexier than pregnancy. A man chose you, out of all the women on earth to share DNA with and make another human.

That's special. That really is something to be happy about. Plenty of women can't find a man, or can't fall pregnant so whenever you're feeling like life is just shit, think about how lucky you are, how loved you are, and how, right now inside your body, a bond of love more powerful than the fabric of the universe has begun to form. With every breath and every positive thought it grows stronger and stronger.

You're lucky. You're very lucky. I am thankful every day for the gifts I've been given. Some people will never get to know the boundless love I am surrounded with every single day. You will. If you already have children you know what I'm talking about.

Will I miscarry?

Let's bump this myth on the head right now. If exercise made you miscarry, then earth would be unpopulated. The mechanics of human pregnancy and birth are the same as for other mammals.

Wild animals don't have the luxury of choice, they have to run, jump, climb and swim. There's no coffee shop for them to sit around *relaxing* with their girlfriends under the premise of 'exercise may harm the baby'.

I would go as far as to say that lack of exercise is worse for your baby. Exercise promotes blood flow. Bloodflow in the body is like rain, it cleans everything out. It flushes toxins and grime and fat out of the system.

Keeping your bloodflow steady, because you don't want to harm the baby is like having a stagnant water system because you're worried it might flood.

I think that the confusion lies in the type of exercise. Exercise can be a stress. A physical stress, if you do exercise that stresses you. High intensity exercise, like sprinting in the heat of the day is just stupid, especially if you've spent the last 10 years sedentary.

Going for a jog in the cool of the day, while listening to your favourite tunes will not only make you feel great, it will help flush out the aftermath of the hormones flowing through your system.

See, it just comes down to common sense. If your body is used to exercise, keep doing it. If you're new to exercise, don't start doing burpees, crossfit and hill sprints.

I used to think that exercise would harm my baby, but when I thought about it I just laughed. If a baby in the stomach was so fragile that we couldn't even exercise with it, how on earth do so many women around the world still have healthy babies with physical jobs? How do antelope breed under the pressure of continuous predatory attack?

Light and Heavy

When it comes to exercise, use common sense. And don't pay too much attention to your trimesters, you'll just confuse yourself. One of the greatest lessons I've got from childbirth is that the baby will come when the baby is ready. There is nothing you can do to bring it on, if it just wants to stay.

Sharny, some things in life, you just can't control...

It's the same for trimesters. I don't believe that they are important. Because there is no distinguishing physical change from trimester to trimester. I think that physically, there are only two phases to pregnancy. I call them light and heavy.

"Light" is how you feel at the first part of the pregnancy. It really is relative, and cannot be quantified, because when compared to not being pregnant, you still feel heavy. But compared to the last part of pregnancy, it feels light.

So all I can say is that you are in the "light" phase until you feel really heavy. And this heaviness actually happens nearly overnight. It's like a changing of the guard. While the trimesters slip by unnoticed, light to heavy is an event. One day, you're feeling like you're pregnant, the next, you feel like you are carrying a child. There is a distinct feeling of separation.

In the light phase, you feel like you and baby are one, but in heavy, you can distinguish between yourself and baby. When you exercise, you feel heavy. Coordination is a lot harder, because like a huge set of boobs (you probably have those now too), your belly moves to it's own rhythm.

Until you were heavy, running felt like it did before you were pregnant, except that you had a belly. Once you hit heavy, running just feels awkward. Your hips don't seem to feel aligned, you feel like a duck trying to waddle, and to top it off, you have this giant bouncy gut, pulling your centre of gravity forward.

When you get to the 'heavy' stage, you'll know it. It's unmistakeable.

There is no set date that the heavy stage happens, it could be a week before birth or it could be a few months. It depends on your genetics and your exercise history. There is no set date, and no way of extending the light phase. So like I had to learn, just go with it.

There are some things in this world you can't control, Sharny…..

But the exciting news is that until you are heavy, pretty much all the exercise you were capable of doing before pregnancy is still acceptable. You'll just be slower, like anyone who has a weight strapped to their stomach and a passenger taking your blood flow.

All sports are OK, as long as there is no risk of bumping or directly hurting your belly. So I wouldn't continue with that UFC career until after the baby was born, but by all means kick the bag!

Sports or activities where you risk falling over are probably best avoided, like water skiing. I'd be wary of exercises that require a high level of balance, because your body can get a little off, once again on account of the extra weight.

Dancing, swimming, running, touch football, tennis, squash and the like are all fine, as long as you listen to your body, and know that you have limits. Obviously no diving for the ball, or getting way too competitive. While you are pregnant, get used to the idea that you won't be your usual competitive self. It's ok to lose, in fact, play for fun, not for a result.

Just listen to your body and your baby. Your intuition is very, very strong and I've had times where I felt like it was OK to do something like hill runs, and then there have been days where I just felt that doing pushups was not going to be good. I liked to believe it was my baby talking to me, but whatever it is, I made sure I listened. Err on the side of caution.

Once you're heavy though, everything feels like running through sand. It's just harder. So once you're heavy, just find things that don't get you frustrated. Like I said before, choose exercises that make you happy. Sign up for a pregnancy yoga class. Go for long walks while you talk or sing to your baby. Ride a bike, go for a swim. All these low impact exercises are great for keeping the body's vitality up.

Some things that doctors recommend you avoid include tummy exercises. Duh. And lifting anything above your head. The reason you don't want to lift things above your head is that your blood pressure had dropped a little. Your heart is working hard, because it's pumping blood around for you, as well as to your placenta. It's working overtime even when you're doing nothing active. So when you do something like lift your arms above your head, you may find that you go a little faint. Don't faint. It's not worth it.

Laying on your back when you're heavy is not ideal either, because the artery that supplies blood to your lower body runs along your spine, laying on your back will sometimes allow the baby to push and squash this artery. Not cool to have blood flow to your lower half blocked. But don't worry; it's not something that goes by unnoticed.

As always, be sensible and observe my golden rule. Do only what makes you happy.

Getting a good sleep

You'll find that sleeping on your back is all but impossible anyway. I like to lie on a full length pillow. I put one leg over the pillow, put my belly into the pillow and tuck one boob on each side of the pillow. Absolute sleeping bliss.

Sleep is another one of those happy serums you can take to ensure a joyful birth experience. Find a way to make yourself sleep well and deep, and you'll have half the birth problems sorted.

Here are my tips for getting an empowering nights' sleep.

Go to the toilet before you go to bed. Even if you've just gone to the toilet. Your insides are being squashed by your little cherub, so your bladder becomes as unreliable as a puppy.

Go to sleep early. You'll need to train yourself for early nights because of early mornings. After this baby is born, you'll forget what a sleep in felt like.

Shower before bed. Some people like to shower in the morning, but I found showering before bed just relaxes and prepares the body for a blissful nights sleep.

Don't play on your phone. Deadshitting is what Julius calls it. Scrolling down the newsfeed for kilometers. Scientists have proven that bright white light, just like from a screen, interferes with our circadian rhythm. In short, you can confuse your body into believing that it is wake time.

I know this is all but impossible for most of us, but if you get into bed before dusk, the changing light somehow makes the ensuing sleep one of the deepest, most relaxing ones you'll ever experience in your life.

Resolve all arguments before you go to your room. Your room is your sanctuary, your happy place. You'll spend a lot of time here with baby in the first few weeks, so you want to program yourself into *knowing* it is a happy place.

Write down a to do list for tomorrow. You've probably noticed your once reliable brain has been letting you down. It's called baby brain. I use the reminders function on my phone, because I'd even forget where I put the piece of paper with the list on it.

Put your phone into flight mode. Not only are messages, emails and phone calls distracting in the night, but there is enough published data on the dangers of short wave radio signals to make me worried about leaving a mini microwave next to my bed with an unborn child in my womb.

Have sex or masturbate. I've said it before, orgasms are like sleeping pills. Except that you can't overdose on orgasms. You made a baby through making love, and I find there is nothing more beautiful and relaxing than falling asleep entwined in your husband after a passionate lovemaking session.

And don't worry, you won't harm the baby. I was worried about this, but even the deepest penetration won't be able to enter the cervix because until you are ready to birth, the entrance is as tight as a bum hole, and behind it is a thick mucus plug that protects the baby from anything getting through.

Have all your jobs done. If you're a happy go lucky kind of girl who just goes with the flow of life, washing clothes when you've run out or leaving dishes until tomorrow, now's the time to change. A routine is essential to keeping sanity once your baby is born, and like any other habit, it's easier to create without the distraction of a baby wanting to be breastfed. Going to sleep knowing the house is clean and everything in order makes for pleasant dreams.

Exercise. If you feel like your sleep is restless, it may be because your body feels like it isn't doing enough to warrant a deep repairing sleep. Sleep is the time that the body recovers from the day of activity. If you haven't done anything active, you may find that your body doesn't give you that sleep you want. If this is the case, make sure you do some kind of exercise the following day – you'll be surprised at how good your sleep can be.

A final note on exercise before I talk about the single greatest pregnancy exercise. You *will* lose condition and you *will* gain weight. Exercise and eat so that you limit that fitness loss and weight gain to an acceptable level. Don't overdo it, just think about it like this:

In less than 9 months, you'll have had the baby and will no longer have a limiter on your exercise intensity (other than time). You're pregnant for 9 months, but you have your baby for up to 20 years. Little habits now, can make a huge difference in a few months time. Believe me, you'll look back on these few months and wonder how you ever thought it could have been difficult.

Squat

You see those posters around social media with a girl who looks like she's smuggling basketballs in her pants and the caption reads "yep, she squats." Most people actually believe that you'll get a big butt from squatting.

I'll take that back a step. Most people believe that a fat ass is sexy, because it is a sign of hard work. Well I can tell you from personal experience that a fat ass is a fat ass because of a fat attitude.

No amount of squatting will make an arse look fat. It will lift a droopy arse, but it certainly won't make it blow out like a pie. I know. When I was fat, I had a flat stomach, and a sexy ass. It was huge and round and bounced when I walked. In tights, I'd be today's version of perfect.

That was until I took my tights off and the 'squatters butt' looked more accurately like a Cheesy McButt – the place I stored my fries and cokes. You know how when you wash a pillow, it comes out all lumpy and uncomfortable?

A squatters arse is the same. All big and beautiful in the pants, but when they come off, it just looks uncomfortable. And I could fool people, except that the pizza topping that was my arse had slipped down to nearly my knees. A fair bit of it was pooled up around my knees.

Even in a bikini, in the right light and a forgiving angle, I could have a photo that says "yep, she squats" but that would require complete relaxation of the cheek muscles, or like pulling a face, you'd see the illusion shattered – like a horror movie. Smooth and round, then BAM! Dented and cloudy.

"Yep, she squats."

Just another misleading fitness trend, covering up the eating habits by saying that she squats. Next we'll see a girl with a spongy gut saying "yep, she situps" or tuckshop arms saying "yep, she tricep extensions."

The only good to come out of this lie is that it's now acceptable for women to squat. Previously we thought we'd get a man body from squatting, so we avoided it. Instead doing about a million lunges.

But for pregnancy, there is no exercise more important than the squat.

Firstly, a squat is a very efficient way of exercising. You can exercise nearly every muscle in your entire body with one movement. Because of this, your heart and lungs have to work very hard to move oxygen around. The strain on your cardiovascular system is enough to keep you fit, without straining your nervous system.

You can strain your nervous system if you want to. This is what creates adaptation, or change. But I'd advise against it because that change comes as a result of hormone releases. Straining your nervous system is stressful.

You have enough hormones flowing through your body that adding in some stress hormones is unnecessary. So just keep your squats light so that you can work your heart and lungs without stressing you out.

The second reason you want to squat is because it puts pressure on your vagina and forces you to exercise your pelvic floor. The deeper you go in your squat, the more you're going to feel like it's going to fall out. If you start squatting early in your pregnancy, you'll never feel this and you'll bounce back after birth with a strong pelvic floor.

It's a lot harder to strengthen a pelvic floor after you've injured it, than it is to make it strong and supple before you give birth, preventing injury. This does come with a warning though, if you are reading this book in the last trimester, don't start squatting if it gives you the feeling of falling out.

You can do leg presses in the gym, or do lunges. A heavy baby on a weak pelvic floor is not a good feeling. To strengthen your pelvic floor, the best exercise is to stop your pee while it is in full flow. I also recommend that while you have sex, to play tug-of-war with your husband's penis. You try to hold it in you like a clamp, and he tries to pull it out. It's a lot more fun that stopping your pee.

The third reason you want to squat is because the squat position is one of the best positions for birthing, simply because you have gravity working *with* your contractions. A birth can last a few hours, so if you've got a lot of squats under your belt, you'll breeze through it. If you can, try to avoid your first deep squat being during labour. That's like your first run being an ultramarathon.

Which brings me to the fourth point.

Squat because it is the equivalent of running training for a marathon. Birthing is a full body experience. It's important that you are prepared for it, and know how to breathe while pushing.

The easiest way to describe giving birth well vs badly is like doing a poo – one where you relax and let it out, or where you force it out by squeezing like little children do.

When training for a marathon, you'll be preparing the body by ensuring that it can run with as little effort as possible. You don't want to be lumbering down the road like an elephant, you want to glide over the surface. Birth is the same. Don't force that baby out like a big poo. Breathe it out and go with the flow of your body's movements.

This is important. Your body flows on it's own during birth; millions of years of evolution has childbirth in your DNA. It's what every mammal knows how to do by instinct. You may not believe it now, but when the time comes, your body will take over. It will do everything on it's own – so go with the flow. Let it run the show. For you, it's just an adventure you're going on. A chance to experience the delicate power of nature first hand. It's truly amazing.

Use your squats to practice your breathing. If you can breathe independently of your squat movement, your birth should be a breeze!

Curing morning sickness

Early in the morning, you can barely raise your head. Inside your stomach feels like you've eaten roadkill. You can't even imagine eating anything. Sound familiar?

Well it is. And it's not what you think.

Morning sickness is very similar to a food hangover. You know when you eat the whole buffet and wind up regretting it the next day. Your stomach hurts and your eyes feel itchy. Your mouth tastes like an ashtray.

In the first 4 pregnancies, I was a basket case - I'd dread going to bed because I knew I was going to be sooooo sick in the morning. This time, when I felt it coming on, I decided to see if I could in fact stop it altogether. I did... and so can you!

To cure my morning sickness, I first had to look at what made the morning sickness worse.

PROBLEM 1: NOT EATING RIGHT.

If I had one of those days where I didn't eat right, meals were badly timed or skipped, I'd guarantee a horrible morning the next day, which would in turn cause me to roll into another day of not eating right.

Solution: control your meals as a matter of priority. Look at all the things that are getting in the way of you eating, then fast forward to tomorrow and you'll see that all those things will be so much easier without morning sickness.

PROBLEM 2: GOING TO BED FULL

I actually discovered this after birth number 4, eating a big meal before bed feels comfortable and normal (or is that expected). But every time I do it, I feel tired and heavy in the morning. I can only assume that it is because the body needs movement to move food down the pipes, so a big meal sitting in the stomach just stays there overnight. Morning sickness kind of feels like you've eaten something that has gone off. Combine this with a meal that has been sitting undigested in your gut for 8 hours and you've got a recipe for a hard morning.

Solution: Eat an early dinner. Our kids eat at 5, so we do too. By the time we go to bed the meal has moved past the stomach to where it is needed.

PROBLEM 3: LOW BLOOD SUGAR IN THE MORNING.

Growing a baby inside you requires quite a lot of energy, and blood sugar levels drop steeply in the night, giving the same sick feeling a diabetic has.

Solution: If you wake up for a toilet stop early in the morning (after 1pm), have a shot of my morning sickness smoothie before going back to bed. After a while you'll get used to waking up 30 minutes before you actually have to wake up, just so you can take the shot (and it works miracles).

Morning sickness smoothie: blend half a green apple, a handful kale/spinach leaves, half a cup ice and a small piece of ginger. Leave in the fridge overnight. 30 minutes before you're meant to wake up, have a shot and go back to bed.

PROBLEM 4: STAYING IN BED SICK

I used to lay in bed and spend most of the morning sick. But laying in bed seems to just make it last longer.

Solution: The body needs to know that it's woken up, so immediately upon waking, do some relatively intense exercise (like 50 quick squats, or run around the block). Morning sickness is weird in that you feel like it's getting worse, then just before you're sure you're going to vomit everywhere, it just lifts like the morning fog.

Morning sickness generally tends to be in the first trimester, when you're not even showing, so you don't need to exercise like you're 9 months pregnant. Get up and crush a quick workout. Even if you're feeling a little woozy, kicking your heart rate up does wonders for your morning sickness, and is the best start to the day!

After your workout, finish the rest of the smoothie and enjoy being pregnant, without the sickness.

Combating Cravings

I think cravings and morning sickness kind of go hand in hand. Like alchohol and hangovers. I remember at uni all the boys saying that the best cure for a hangover is another drink. And it worked. Until the next day.

I found that with my first 4 fat-girl pregnancies, I wouldn't be able to eat until lunch time because of morning sickness, at which point I was so hungry that I would begin to crave anything. Ice-cream, chocolate, Mcdonalds fries and all sorts of wonderful concoctions that I knew weren't good for baby.

But I just let them go, because, you know, cravings are my right. I'm pregnant, so I crave things.

I'm not saying cravings don't exist, what I am saying is that many of us use cravings as an excuse to eat crap. In the beginning of this book, I challenged you to use this time of unfiltered thinking to do something productive and good for yourself, because it's expected of you.

Most mums use this time of unfiltered, unjudged time to eat everything they ever wanted. I know I did. "stuff it, I'm pregnant" seemed to be the motto of my day as I did my drive through window pub crawl.

I thought that if I didn't go back to a particular drive through nobody would notice that I had already eaten 6 packets of fries that morning. But I pretended not to care… "Stuff it, I'm pregnant!"

You can do that, there's really nothing stopping you. You'll enjoy it too. I felt so deeply satisfied sitting on the couch watching infomercials with a 4 litre tub of icecream, challenging myself to finish it before it became a milkshake. I'd dip my fries in the icecream or try and suck them up through a straw.

I loved it. Until the next morning. All that junk filled me up, so I couldn't drink water. In the morning, my sickness would be so profound, so heavy, and all the images of me being a total glutton would haunt me as I threw up string fries and milk froth.

I'd swear that I wouldn't do it again. All morning, I'd swear. Then like a heroin addict, I'd find an excuse to get in the car and drive somewhere. My carefully planned route would take me all over town, to most of the fast food joints, then to the supermarket to get supplies.

And I say supplies because I was like a teenager preparing for a weekend in front of the TV. The only groceries were the ones used to cover the rest of the crap in the trolley.

I was a disgrace. And when I finally worked it out, it was too late. After my 4th Baby, I was too big for my frame. I looked like a lawn grub. My skin was shiny all the time because of how stretched it was.

I knew what to do; just change my eating and exercise, but I had two major problems. Firstly, my cravings had become habits. It's very, very hard to break a habit. And secondly, I had a business to run, while looking after 3 kids under 3.

If you think resisting cravings is hard, I can tell you beating them after birth, when you have no sleep and no energy and your body is coming back together is all but impossible. Do yourself a favour and don't give in to them.

A moment on the lips, can mean a lifetime on the hips.

And here's how to logic it out. Some women crave washing powder or glass. Glass isn't good for you, so they just don't eat it. Obviously. This is proof then, that cravings aren't irresistible.

So if you're craving something that you know isn't good for you, use the same amount of willpower these women use to avoid glass. You'll thank yourself in the morning when you're not sick, and you'll feel like you've avoided a total disaster once you've had the baby and you don't have to beat cravings that have turned into habits. Habits that have turned into addictions.

You really can do this. Junk food cravings are usually a sign that you are feeling trapped and want to do something out of control. Go and do something self affirming. Sunbathe naked in the back yard. Go to the beach and read a book, ride a bike, walk through the botanical gardens, have an hour long bath, turn the music up and dance. You still own your life!

Cravings for other things are usually signs that your body is missing something. Chocolate can mean that your body wants more love. Ice means that your body wants more iron. Google is your best friend here. If you are craving something consistently, then look it up!

Don't just give in to them.

Have a plan

The most amazing thing about birth is that you don't have to know what to do. From the moment of your conception, you've been programmed for this.

Animals know this, they can birth multiple babies under a tree on their own. You're no different. Except that you think you can't. Somehow through our evolution, we've decided that birth is a medical emergency.

Obstetricians are emergency doctors. They should step in if there is an emergency. Not control the whole situation. Which brings me to the next section.

My brother in law is a surgeon. I'd like to say he's a new age surgeon, but I don't know any others. I'd venture as far as to say that the anti-medical-bandwagon is similar to the ancient Europeans who thought that black people were demons.

They had just never met one.

But, in the face of it, I'll say that to them, he's a new age surgeon. When I ask him a medical question, he assesses first whether he can help, by consulting the encyclopedia of medical knowledge that he has in his head. Then tells me if he can help, or if not.

If he can't help, he refers me to someone who can. A lot of these issues are not surgical, but because he is Doctor Kieser, I ask his advice on everything medical.

His response is always "My tools of trade are a script pad and a scalpel. My answers will always be dictated by my training. Remember that if you cut something out, you can't put it back, and if you drug it, there may be side effects."

My opinion of natural birth is that the experts go in this order.

Your body.

Midwife.

Surgeon.

Medics know this. Of all of my kids, I have only needed medical intervention once. And it was my fault. I'll elaborate a bit for you.

Your body knows what to do via genetic code. If you let it be and just relax, most of the work will be done for you. All of the decision-making will be done for you.

If your body needs something of you, it will tell you. As long as you are calm and prepared for the messages, your body will tell you.

A midwife is trained to read the signs. A midwife knows more about a natural birth than an obstetrician simply because they are in the coal face. They are the ones delivering babies all day long. Obstetricians are great at birth emergencies.

A midwife can only read the signs if you are calm and cooperative.

An obstetrician is not a midwife. An obstetrician is there as an emergency medical back up. It's a good thing if you don't see them during birth. If you do see them, don't panic either – they are just checking that everything is going well.

You'll notice during birth that there is this chain of command. Your body talks to you and shows signs to the midwife. The midwife relays these signs to the obstetritian.

An obstetritian is there just in case something goes wrong.

Now, before the anti-medical-bandwagon starts up their drum circle, please understand that obstetricians are good people. I know some chiropractors who swear obstetricians are the devil. They're not. They have a duty of care to you and your baby, and will seize control if you have lost it. Which is what happened with my first baby.

I lost control and panicked. The worst thing you can do is panic. As soon as you panic, your bottom end closes up, while the top end continues it's pushing down. Panic is a byproduct of fear. Fear causes birth problems.

Trust that you've got this. Because you do. You've totally got this. But if you don't and you start to lose control, the obstetritian will step in and ensure a safe delivery of your baby.

They look for signs. And one of the first signs that a birth is going to be challenging is a panicky mother. Avoid panic and you'll be fine. But even if you do – be comforted by the fact that a highly skilled, precision trained birth surgeon is there, along with a team of expert midwives to ensure your birth runs smoothly.

There really is no reason to ever panic.

I'm a highly-strung person. Panic has always come naturally to me. Every time I bake a birthday cake, I go into freak out mode. I expected to make it look like this, but it ended up looking like that.

It sounds trivial, but it's more common than you think.

Pregnancy is the same. You may plan on having the home birth with the incense burning and the calming music, but end up giving birth in a car park at the supermarket.

So instead of only planning for the perfect birth, plan for alternative scenarios. It's so much easier to cover off on potential emergency situations before they happen.

Under the pressure of an event, it's much better to consult the plan, than to make decisions. Spend some time now, deciding on how you are going to tackle each of the following decisions:

- Where are you going to give birth?
- If you can't get there, how will you adapt?
- What will you do if the baby is premature?
- How long are you prepared to go over due date before you intervene? How will you intervene?
- What is your plan if the baby is posterior?

- What is your plan if the baby is in breach?

- Who is in charge of talking to the midwives?

- What music are you going to listen to to relax, where is it and what happens if you can't listen to it?

- When the contractions start, how long will you wait until you go to hospital?

- What can your husband do if you begin to panic?

- At what point (under what circumstances) would you want the obstetrician to step in?

- Are you going to use drugs or not? If you are, what are they, when will you take them and how much?

- Are you prepared to have an epidural?

- What clothes are you going to have in a bag for birth?

- Have you got spare clothes in case you wet/soil yours?

- Have you got breast pads and maternity pads?

- Have you installed and checked the baby seat?

- Have you researched all the injections that your baby may get and decided if they will or will not have them?

- Have you done your own research on immunisation and are making an informed decision?

- What are you going to do with your other children? What if you can't do that and they have to come with you?

- Have you prepared any other siblings for the arrival of their new baby brother or sister?

- You may stay in hospital for 5 days, are you prepared for that?

- Is your husband prepared for you to be away from home for 5 days?

- What food will you eat while at the hospital. Who will make it/buy it, and how will you store it there. Hospital food is generally very low in nutrition, cheap crap.

There are literally hundreds of scenarios that could happen with childbirth. I strongly, strongly suggest you sit down with your husband and plan out what will happen in each of them. You may never experience any of them, but it's so much better to decide what to do when you're calm, than to make a decision under pressure.

We've got our plan for each birth, including our action steps in the event of a disaster or emergency. It's not nice to think about it, but it is reassuring to know what you're going to do.

It's kind of like your own first aid course. You never want anything bad to happen, but if it does, at least you know what you're going to do.

I've found that the best thing is to make the decision with your husband, then leave it up to him to be in charge. I want to be fully focussed on listening to my body and enjoying the experience, while he communicates with the midwife and the doctors and anyone else.

There should be nobody in the world that you trust more than your husband. He has your best interest at heart, so trusting him to be the insulation between you and the outside world just makes sense.

And by husband, I mean birth partner. Someone you feel is the best person to be there *for you* during birth. And just like I said before, plan for if your birth partner is not there either.

Sometimes the plan is just coming to terms with the fact that you'll be alright. For me, this was my biggest fear – not having Julius there with me. But when I spent some time thinking about it, running the scenario through my head, I felt confident that I could handle it. I may not like it, but I could handle it.

We live in a different world to our parents and grandparents, where birth was women's business. Gone are the days where the man sits at the pub with his mates while you labour on your own.

I'll let Julius take over from here, because he feels very strongly about it.

The next chapter is for you to read, but more importantly for your husband to read. Having Julius there for my births was the most empowering, reassuring, marriage-strengthening experiences that neither he, nor I, would ever want to have missed.

Father to father

I'll start this by saying any dick can make a baby. But it takes a real man to be a father. I'll extend that to any dick can lure a woman, but it takes a real man to be a husband.

The idea of a real man is a bit muddy, so I'm going to set the record straight here. Any of you pissy, whiny little boys who think that birth is the realm of women only, not only have no balls, but shouldn't consider themselves men.

You know how your back sometimes hurts when you spend too long standing in one place? Imagine that pain for ¾ of a year. Now imagine you can't ever sit down either. That pain is there whether you sit, stand, lie down or even fall asleep. You're not injured, you're just pregnant.

Now imagine that everywhere you go, people are looking at you with judgemental eyes. Everything you eat, and everything you even buy is looked at with disdain.

Now imagine dropping a watermelon out of your pee hole. Not straight away, but in the time it takes to play back to back football games. Barefoot and naked. You can't take a pee break, so you have to piss yourself in front of a crowd. Same with poo. It's going to just fall out of you on it's own.

That's what your wife is going to go through, so if you think you deserve to sit at a pub with your dropkick mates Damo and Davo, I've got something coming for you. Its called a nappy. Because you're a fucking baby. A little bitch boy who should go back to your little bitch boy daddy and suck his fucking nipples. Because he was not man enough to say "I'll be there for you," to your mum.

As men, we love sport and war movies that hail the call "no man left behind," so now's your chance to stand beside your best friend in all the world, the one you chose to serve and protect. Now's your chance to prove that you were worth choosing.

You want bravery, you sit there like an overgrown child playing your Xbox eating yourself to death, believing that you would actually be tough? Well now's your chance, fanny boy. Because what your wife is about to go through, is tougher than anything any man on earth could ever go through. So you better be there for her.

You think you're tough because you swore at someone from inside your car, or you took the rubbish out at night by yourself, or you tackled that big Samoan guy in high school. You've got nothing on what your wife can do. Nothing.

I don't. My wife is ten times the man I am. If we measure manliness by toughness. If we do, then every mother on earth is tougher than even the toughest man.

You fight in the UFC or played Origin? Soft compared to your wife.

I've heard little boy-men saying stupid things like "I just don't wanna see her vagina that way," Boys like this are an embarrassment to men the world over. I pity their wives, because they were fooled into choosing a faggy little boy, who dressed up like a man. It's like the sheep got dressed up in wolf clothing.

That arrogant man-child is going to grow up to be the show dad standing on the sideline yelling at 5 year old kids. Fuck that dad. You don't want to be that dad.

I hear these guys saying things like "I don't think I could ever go near her again after seeing a baby come through there." Well, you don't deserve to go near her ever again you flake.

If that's your opinion and you are too much of a little bitch to be there for your wife, then she should feel like a pedophile every time you come at her with that tiny excuse of a cock again. You're a boy, not a man. Go play toys with your friends, child.

But you're not like that. As soon as my wife fell pregnant, I knew I had to be more manly. I had to get rid of every vestibule of boyhood and become a man. Because only men can raise children right. Boys can't raise children. Men can.

So you have two choices right now. You can admit that you don't have the courage to be a man, and therefore submit to your wife and go under her care as your mother. Sounds nice and I know a lot of men who grew up to have a second mother. If that's you then that's cool, you've chosen to remain a boy. But boys don't get to have sex with their mothers. So don't ever complain to me about your shitty sex life. Your wife is probably embarrassed about you.

Boys don't get to have sex with their mothers, men get to make love to their wives. If you're a boy, you don't deserve to taste the sweet nectar of your wife's loving. You deserve a lifetime of dick in hand, fantasising about what could have been... If you weren't such a coward. It's why boys bitch about their shitty sex lives, while real men make love to a goddess.

And that's all we really want from our wives, right? We want them to be our own private porn starlet. Our sex goddess. We want to be making love to them thinking "holy shit, nobody on earth is as lucky as me!"

I'm willing to bet my career that inside every woman is a sexual goddess just aching to escape. But she needs a man to rescue her from her girlhood. A man. Be that man.

The way the male population has interpreted woman's equality has bred the wrong kind of man. We've swung from ignorant-man-troll to over-sensitive-lady-boy. Be man enough to stand in the middle. Strong enough to be your wife's rock, but sensitive enough to understand her needs. Your body is her hammer, your chest is her pillow and your heart is her best friend.

Woah. I think imay have gone a bit overboard there. The keyboard warrior in me was in full flight and I just didn't want to stop him. All that aggression... what? I think I need to go eat some carbs. It's in a book, so we'll call it poetic license. I must be compensating for something...

Here's the truth. Until I met my wife, my life was peppered with bad decisions and regrets. I was a constant source of disappointment for my parents. I only ever cared about myself.

Then one day I made the commitment to marry Sharny. To care for and protect someone other than myself. I didn't take it lightly and the weight of that responsibility is very important to me. I chose to give my emotional, mental and physical strength to her.

When we decided to have kids, it was a decision. I *chose* to then care for and protect each and every one of them for the rest of my life. I swore, before each of them was conceived that I would be there for them. I would do everything I could to be there for them when they needed me... Everything I could.

That decision lead me to wondering about what events in their lives they *would* need me. Birthing a baby is one of those moments. Not just for the child, but for your wife. She is in the most vulnerable state she will ever be in. I decided that NOTHING would get in the way of me being there for her.

The impact of that decision has filtered down through the rest of my life. I wasn't just a witness to the miracle of childbirth, I was involved in it. I was a teammate.

Before the baby, you're husband and wife. After you go through a birth together, you become one. When people go through something big together, they become so much closer than they ever thought possible. It's like that, but more powerful.

After being there for the birth, I realised how much I was actually needed. Not only then, but in the next few days and it got me thinking that fathers who go out drinking to celebrate the birth of their child are missing out on one of the most profound experiences of their lives.

Not only that, but they are setting one helluva low standard of family living. Going drinking instead of looking after my wife and new baby would be a regret I just couldn't live with.

There are so few profound memories in a human life, birth being one of them. I wouldn't want to get to the end of my life, look back and see that I had missed the opportunity to be there for the people I swore to protect.

I chose this wife, and I chose to make this family with her. I will never put myself ahead of them. I chose to be a husband and I chose to be a father. Choices that I certainly don't take lightly. Being a father is not an award, it's a privilege.

So, here's my list of rules for myself, for being the best husband around birth time. Use some of my rules, add some of your own, discard all of mine, but have a list. It'll certainly help solidify your commitment to yourself and your family.

Firstly, finances are not your only role. That's like sponsoring your mates football team and not playing. You've got to play the game to enjoy it. Life is the game, don't miss it all and then think you can buy it back.

You're breeding a best friend with your best friend. You're not on the outside looking in, this baby will grow up to be a man one day, in which case you want to show him how to be one, or it's going to be a woman one day, in which case you want to be the benchmark of manliness for her future husband. Get involved – you've got a best friend coming if you choose it.

Don't become a fat pig. Your wife is going through hormonal hell. She's going to want to eat some particularly disgusting shit. Don't you give in to her cravings. Doing that is a cycle, because she'll think it's the only thing you enjoy together.

Stay as fit and healthy as you can. You giving up on your body is like a big neon sign to her that you just don't give a shit about her anymore. Junk food and beer are more important. Make her proud to be on your arm. You want a sexy wife? Be sexy to her.

Pregnancy is a team effort. There are things that you can do to make it easier on your beautiful wife. Once it's done, you want to feel like you achieved it together as a team, rather than just "my wife did it all."

You won't fully understand what's going on, but you can help. Imagine trying to shit out a concrete pylon. At the same time, someone is papercutting the head of your dick and someone else is swinging two hammers at your balls. Birth is painless compared to that. And your wife will do it with little fuss. Don't be fooled by how easy she's making it look – she's a warrior.

One of the biggest things you can do to help is to be present. Like a knight. In the old days, women of stature had their own personal knight who would silently protect them. Their role was to be there for the woman at all times. A physical presence, a guard against harm. Your presence is like that for her. Be present.

Be romantic. Trimester two, you'll have a wild sex goddess if you play your cards right – you'll have the best sex of your life. Not even the wildest drunk nubile porn star can compare to the sexual perfection of your wife in tri 2.

Don't listen to your mates unless they are real men. Your mates are boys who don't understand what it is to be a man. They're like school yard children talking about girl's germs.

Birth is like getting front row seats to a grand final that your wife is playing in, then being invited to lift the trophy. It's a once in a lifetime opportunity. Accept the challenge with both hands and see the miracle of childbirth first hand.

Be as hands on as you can. Doctors are tough people with fantastic empathy. Birth is not women's business. Do you think Doctors are only women? My brother is one of the toughest men on earth. At age 12 he walked into a forest in the middle of the night to investigate some particularly terrifying screaming. He was barefoot and armed with just a rock. He grew up to become a doctor. The type of doctor who with the gentlest of whispers can calm a terrified child. The type of doctor who can reset bones after terrible trauma. He would never shy away from blood. You don't want him to be the man whispering gently to your wife, do you?

I promise you that the depth of love you feel for your wife will multiply infinitely after you share this experience with her. She will feel the same for you.

One thing you do have is the capacity to diffuse a stressful situation. You're going to need all of those powers when you're in the hospital surrounded by women. Midwives will look at you like you don't belong. Take ownership of the situation and calm their nerves. It's not their fault, they've seen far too many lady-boy husbands come in with their wives and end up just getting in the way.

Be prepared for everything - learn about all the shitty things that could happen and have a plan. Don't tell your wife about anything that could scare her. Just tell her the plan if you have to. You are the police officer/fireman/ambo.

Be the insulation for your wife when she gives birth. You're the cotton wool that wraps her and protects her from the outside world. On the outside of the cotton wool is a sheet of iron. Only you get to talk to her, and you convey messages from her to the midwives and doctors and family and friends… You're the steady one. You're the man.

Go with the flow. Your wife has, in her genetic code, the capacity to birth this baby naturally on her own. But we live in a pretty messed up world, with experts on every corner trying to get you to spend your money with them. You really don't need anyone. Just go with the flow, and at all times remember that you are your wife's husband. You are the father of this child. And this is the greatest adventure you could ever dream of going on, with the one person on earth you adore above everyone else.

Don't worry if you don't fall in love straight away - she's had 9 months. Most people say that you'll fall in love with your child straight away. You might, but my experience is that once the little milk guzzler starts smiling at you, you'll know what love for a child is. There will be a point that you suddenly feel insignificant and afraid, because the world is so dark and terrible a place for this innocent little soul. You'll swear silently then that you will be it's protector for life (and you'll mean in – in that first smile, you give your life to your child).

Having a boy is not better than having a girl. They're both beautiful and unique and wonderful. It's old fashioned and stupid to wish for a boy. Real men raise wonderful daughters.

Changing a little girl's nappy is easy – it's just a credit card swipe. Changing a boy is harder, but you've got the same gear, so you'll work it out.

Be the man on the phone – take calls and answer messages and book people in for visits. But only when your wife feels comfortable. Read her body language, when she looks like she's had enough, get the people out.

When your mother in law rocks up smelling like a bag of pot pourri, be a man and turn her away. Strong smells stress babies out. Babies strongest sense is their sense of smell, so it's your job to turn people away.

There are no such thing as women's jobs and men's jobs. Unless it's breastfeeding.

Enjoy it. Whether you like it or not, you're already a man. You just have to be one, for your wife, your child and especially for the lost little boys out there, dressed up as men. And lastly for us real men. There aren't many around so it would be good to have a few more. We'll notice each other across a carpark as we unload the pram or change a nappy in the boot and we'll smile, because we know. In this world of oestro-men, we're in good company.

A note from your husband

Hi honey. I know this time is all about the baby, but I wanted to take a moment out of your day to tell you that I love you. Not just say the words, I want you to know that I truly love you.

Pretty soon, we'll have a little baby, who will take all the focus off us. It wasn't long ago that it was just me. Then, in a whirlwind of rightness, it became you and me. We've been you and me for a while now, enough for me to sometimes feel comfortable in it. To appear to take you for granted.

This is not the case. There may be days or weeks that go by without me showing you affection of telling you that I love you. You may feel it's unloving of me, but it's a man's way of showing that he loves you. I'm a problem solver. If it's fixed, I leave it alone. If I built a car from scratch, I'd love it every day and remember every detail of the journey, but I wouldn't feel the need to clean it every day. That doesn't mean I love it less or have forgotten about it.

It means that it is perfect just the way it is. Like you. I don't shower you with gifts and kisses and compliments, because you're perfect. I really want you to know that.

And now, with this pregnancy, you've taken this feeling of love and changed it. Enhanced it. I thought that love was what it was, until you fell pregnant.

When we first met, and the reason I love you is because you inspire me to be better at life, every day. You inspired me to be better than I thought I could have ever been.

In time, that love has not faded, but become a part of me. Like a scar, but a good one. I can remember the passionate love we had when we first met, and I through familiarity have appeared to become complacent. In actual fact I am still just trying to live up to the person I promised you I would be.

But with your glow, I feel that all consuming love again. I can't stop thinking about you. I see you now, as though it's the first time again. I look at every part of you, like the curve of your shoulders or the colour of your eyes like I'm seeing you again for the first time.

I am falling in love with you again. Which is logically impossible, but that's the only thing I can compare it to. It would be more accurate to say then, that I am falling in love with you, deeper.

I feel once again that drive to be better. Better for you, better to you. I feel lucky that you, the most beautiful woman on earth could have chosen me, above all the other men in this world.

And when I say lucky, I really feel it. It gives me a weird bumping feeling in my chest and a lightness to my stomach when I think about you and your choice to call me the father of our child..

Our child.

Even saying "our" child gives me shivers. I was just a boy, trying to make a girl love him. Now, I've got the most holy of all confirmations that my tactics had worked. You're carrying our baby in your stomach.

Our baby.

It was you and me, and now it's going to be you, me and baby. Please know that as a boy, I thought my tactics were to lure you, to capture your heart. I now know that they weren't. They were to free you, to allow yourself to be you. Because you are perfect, just the way that you are.

I really want to give you the freedom to be whatever type of mother you want to be. You know, better than any expert, what type of mother will be best for our baby. I want you to know that whatever you choose, I will support you unfalteringly. I will be your shield and your sword.

I want you to know that even though the stereotypical father doesn't show excitement or emotion, I am over the moon. We're being given full custody of a helpless, beautiful, perfect little baby. I hope for their sake they look more like you than me.

I hope that they get your eyes, your zest for life and your energy. They'll be perfect so I'm sure they will. I hope that I can teach them how to throw a ball, catch a fish, cook the perfect steak and change a tyre.

Above all else I hope I can show them how much I love you.

I want them to be proud of me, the same way that I want you to be proud of me. I want to be the best father in the world. And that starts with being the best husband. I know I've got it in me; it pulses in the pit of my soul when I think about you and this baby.

You're amazing, but I can't find the words to describe it to you, I feel clumsy. Words don't come easily to me, so I hope you notice my actions.

Your changing body is beautiful. You may think it looks puffy and veiny and gross (your words). But that's probably because you are still seeing yourself as a girl. I prefer you as a woman than as a girl.

Pretty soon we'll be birthing this baby. I want to be there. Not just as a spectator, but as a teammate. A partner. We're going to do this together. That sub-current of panic that you feel, forget it. I'm here for you and I want to take some of your load, physical, mental and emotional.

We're making a best friend together. I want to be there for every important milestone in their lives, starting with birth.

By the time this baby is ready to come out, I'll have a plan for every scenario. You don't need to know them unless you want to, I just want you to relax in the fact that I have a plan. All you need worry about is enjoying the experience and connecting with your baby so that he/she comes into the world safely and calmly.

Don't stereotype me, I want the challenge of changing a nappy or bottle feeding. I am a man, and I'm not afraid of poo or crying babies. I will also be the king of burping. That is what it is. I've been good at it since I was a boy and I'm going to teach this little munchkin how to do it. Wind is nothing to me, just a challenge accepted.

First it was you, then it was you and me. Now it's going to be you, me and the kids. But even though we will always be a family, I want you to know that the family is nothing without our love. I know this and I will work on it.

Our love for each other is the most sacred gift we can give to this child. I promise that I will do a better job at showing affection, leaving my comfort zone to gently pat you on the bum in public or hold your hand at events. I will show the world that this man puts his love for his wife, and his family ahead of all else. Just like I will be your castle walls at birth, I will be the castle walls for this family forever.

I searched the world and all my life for you. I now give myself to you. To protect you, to respect you and to love you.

I will love you forever

Practice makes perfect

Just like any sport, or event, it's a good idea to practice. No, it's a GREAT idea.

You obviously can't practice contractions, but you can practice nearly everything else. Muscle memory. Just like your plan for birthing scenarios, it's comforting to know that you can do the things you should be doing.

Like breathing. There are two styles of breathing that certainly help ease the passage of your baby. Instead of doing short, raspy little breaths, you should be trying to breath down into your womb.

Try it now. Take a deep breath into your lungs, now use your tummy to get even more breath in. Hold it for a second, and breathe it out slowly. The whole time, visualise the air getting to your womb. Oxygenating it, relaxing it.

You should feel like the breath goes into your mouth, down into your lungs and out through your belly button. The out breath should take around 3 times as long as the in breath. Try it a few times now to get the hang of it. You should feel really, really relaxed after about 10 breaths. Your body should be much more oxygenated and you'll feel focussed, but calm.

This type of breathing is paramount to a calm birth. It requires steady concentration, but if all you need to focus on in the final stages of birth is your breathing, then it is quite easy. This is why it is so important to have a birth partner there with you. Let them answer questions, you just focus on your breathing.

The next thing you need to practice is visualising your vagina opening from the inside. Like a rosebud turning into a flower. It goes a long way to relaxing you if you just picture a rosebud opening into a flower. From the inside out, rather than just stretching. Look on youtube for a timelapse video of a rosebud opening if you can't picture it in your head.

I would go as far as to say that every time you go to the toilet, you should visualise the rose bud, while you do your deep breathing. Toilet time is a great time to do it because you have to go to the toilet at least once a day, and you'll get good feedback. When you feel like you can breathe a poo out with ease, you'll know that you're more than ready for birthing.

Next, find what relaxes you. What music totally calms you down. I'm a fan of Tony O'Connor – his music is beautiful and relaxing. Enya and Adele are other good options.

Every night before bed, I'd suggest you put the relaxing music on, breathe yourself to a completely relaxed state and drift off to sleep. My best births were in a trance like state. You know when you're completely and utterly relaxed, like near the end of a delicious massage? You're awake, but drifting in and out of half sleep? That's the state I like to birth in.

Remember that you body knows what to do unconsciously. You've just got to try and get yourself out of the way.

What is very helpful is that the music you listen to to relax you for birth is being listened to by your baby in your tummy. So when he or she comes out and is restless, the same music will remind him/her of how relaxed mummy was, so they will relax too. Remember that

we're imprinting our emotions onto the baby in utero. Complete relaxation is an emotion. Your baby will feel that from you and respond in kind.

Your husband can help you to get fully relaxed too. Ask him to tickle your back with the back of his fingers, tracing them up and down and across your back. Up into your hair and down your arms. He wants to help, and this is one of the best ways to help. Only he knows how to relax you completely. It will also give him something to do while you are birthing, that will allow him to be close to you. Allow him to be your insulation. Allow him to be your teammate, whispering in your ear, reminding you to breathe deeply and telling you how well you are doing.

Get him to tickle your back in whatever positions you feel most comfortable birthing in. I found birthing with my knees on the ground and arms resting on a chair (or the edge of a birth pool) to be most comfortable, so we practiced that.

The final thing I'd recommend is to stretch your perineum. It's the muscle at the opening of your vagina that gets stretched at birth. To do it yourself, sit in the bottom of the shower and place your thumb into your vagina and push down to stretch it toward the shower floor.

Do that until you feel like you don't need to any more (maybe every night for 2 weeks), then enlist the help of your husband. Lay on your back on the bed, and practice your breathing. Get him to put the first knuckle of his thumb into your vagina and press down toward the bed slowly until it stretches. Breathe until the pain subsides and ask him to stretch it further. Each day you do it, you'll find that it gets more and more supple.

Having a supple perineum will help to prevent tears and will help with keeping a strong pelvic floor after birth.

If you practice the things you need to do for a comfortable natural birth, you'll be doing more than 90% of birthing mothers out there and will therefore prevent the number one birth problem. Fear.

You're ready

So, after flipping through a whole bunch of subjects and topics, we come to the end. Just like pregnancy, you have to move on. But before you do, I really want you to know that you're perfect. You have been chosen above every other person on earth, to be wholly and fully responsible for this little soul growing in your tummy.

You wouldn't have been chosen if that little cherub didn't believe in you. Birth is a wonderful, empowering experience that I hope you and your husband get to experience together. But don't forget that there is another person who will be present and helping in this event.

They'll actually be doing a lot more work that you will. I'm talking about your baby. When they decide it's time, then it's time. You will get to experience the power of a child's purpose. Nothing on earth will change their minds. Once they've decided it's time to come out and cuddle you, they're coming out.

I want you to take strength from that experience. If a little, helpless baby can control everything like that, imagine what you could do if you harnessed the purpose you were born with.

You've been chosen for a reason. I think it's more than just because you'll be a good mother. I think it's because you are a good human. You have good in you and the power to change the world for the better.

In your tummy, you hold the future of humanity. You control the future.

I'm proud of you and I know you'll do what is right and just in this world of chaos. I know that you will give this little soul the start in life it deserves, so that one day, when they leave the nest, they will do so without hangups or hindrances. They will be powerful beyond measure because you made sure you showed them what real freedom is.

Freedom… Is Joy.

Talk to us!

We'd love to hear from you, please let us know if and how this book has helped you. Just shoot us a quick email at

sharnyandjulius@sharnyandjulius.com

Thankyou for taking the time to read our book!

Sharny and Julius Kieser

You can also follow us on social media by searching:

sharnyandjulius

The Kiesers